Traditional Chinese Treatment for Andropathy

Chief-Editor: Hou Jinglun
Editor: Zhao Xin, Li Guohua

Academy Press [Xue Yuan]

First Edition 1997
ISBN7 – 5077 – 1339 – 3

Traditional Chinese Treatment for Andropathy
Chief – Editor: Hou Jinglun
Editor: Zhao Xin Li Guohua

Published by
Academy Press [Xue Yuan]
11 Wanshoulu Xijie, Beijing 100036, China

Distributed by
China International Book Trading Corporation
35 Chegongzhuang Xilu, Beijing 100044, China
P. O. Box 399, Beijing, China

Printed in the People's Republic of China

Preface

Traditional Chinese Medicine and Pharmacology(TCMP) has a long history. It summed up abundant clinical experience in the struggle against diseases. It has formed an integrated, unique and first of all, a scientific system of both theory and clinical practice. On the fundamental principle of 'Zhengtiguannian'(Wholism) and 'Bianzhenglunzhi'(Treatment of the same disease with different therapies). TCM treatment is effective for various kinds of diseases with few side-effect taken. At present, a great upsurge in learning, practising and studying TCM is just in the ascendant. For the benefit of people of all countries, we edited this book in order to promote the spread of TCM all over the world.

In this book, we introduced comprehensively TCM treatment for commonly encountered male diseases and therapies such as drug therapy, acupuncture and moxibustion, Qigong, massage, dietic therapy, etc. are suggested accordingly. This series is the best for those foreign friends who want to learn and master traditional Chinese medicine.

May everyone of all nations enjoy a healthy life!

Chief - Editor

Contents

Chapter One	Urinary Infection	(1)
Chapter Two	Mammary Development	(12)
Chapter Three	Acute Glomerulonephritis	(18)
Chapter Four	Chronic Glomerulonephritis	(27)
Chapter Five	Nephrotic Syndrome	(37)
Chapter Six	Urolithiasis	(40)
Chapter Seven	Chronic Prostatitis	(54)
Chapter Eight	Hyperplasia of Prostate	(63)
Chapter Nine	Epididymitis	(72)
Chapter Ten	Tuberculosis of Epididymitis	(76)
Chapter Eleven	Hydrocele of Tunica Vaginalis	(81)
Chapter Twelve	Induration of Penis	(87)
Chapter Thirteen	Balanoposthitis	(90)
Chapter Fourteen	Enuresis	(94)
Chapter Fifteen	Diabetes Insipidus	(101)
Chapter Sixteen	Retention of Urine	(103)
Chapter Seventeen	Chyluria	(107)
Chapter Eighteen	Impotence	(111)
Chapter Nineteen	Male Sterility	(118)
Chapter Twenty	Carcinoma of Kidney, Renal Pelvis and Ureter	(125)
Chapter Twenty-one	Commonly Used Recipes	(136)

Anti-inflammatory and Analgesic Bolus (136)
Anti-inflammatory Pill (137)
Acanthopanax Infusion (138)
Banlong Pill (139)
Baolong Pill (140)
Bolus for Activating Meridians (141)
Bolus for Severe Endogenous Wind-Syndrome (143)
Bolus of Arisaematis (144)
Bolus of Placenta Hominis (146)
Bolus of Precious Drugs (148)
Bolus of Storax (149)
Brain-Invigorating and Kidney-Tonifying Pill (151)
Cardiotonic Pill (152)
Decoction for Activating Blood Circulation (153)
Decoction for Eliminating Dampness and Relieving Rheumatism (155)
Decoction for Hemiplegia (156)
Decoction for Invigorating Spleen and Nourishing heart (157)
Decoction for Invigorating Yang (159)
Decoction for Mild Hemiplegia (160)
Decoction for Removing Blood Stasis in the Chest (162)

Decoction for Sterility	(164)
Decoction for Treating Rheumatism	(165)
Decoction of Bupleuri Adding Os Draconis and Concha Ostreae	(167)
Decoction of Bupleuri and Puerariae for Expelling Evil from Muslces	(169)
Decoction of Cimicifugae and Astragali seu Hedysari	(170)
Decoction of Cinnamomi Aconiti	(172)
Decoction of Cinnamomi, Glycyrrhizae, etc.	(173)
Decoction of Cinnamomi, Paeoniae and Aemarrhenae	(174)
Antipyretic and Antitoxic Bolus	(176)
Bolus of Calculus Bovis for Purging the Heart-Fire	(177)
Bolus of Citri Grandis	(177)
Bolus of Rhei and Eupolyphaga seu Steleophaga	(179)
Bolus of Six Drugs Including Rehmannia	(181)
Bolus of Ten Powerful Tonics	(183)
Cow-bezoar Bolus for Clearing Away Heat of the Upper Part of the Body	(184)
Decoction for Clearing Away Pestilent Factors and Detoxification	(185)
Decoction for Clearing Heat in Ying System	(187)
Decoction for Strngthening Middle Jiao and Benefiting Vital Energy	(188)
Decoction of Arctii for Soothing Muscles	(190)
Decoction of Coptidis for Detoxification	(192)
Decoction of Cinnamomi Adding Cinnamomi	(193)
Decoction for General Antiphlogistic	(195)
Decoction for Purging Liver-fire and Eliminating Dampness	(196)
Golden Lock Bolus for Keep Kidney Essence	(198)
Zaizao Powder	(199)
Powder for Antiphlogosis	(201)
Pill of Six Miraculous Drugs	(203)
Decoction of Phragmitis	(205)
Powder of Lonicerae and Forsythiae	(206)
Powder of Ledebouriellae for Dispersing the Superficies	(208)
White Tiger Decoction	(210)
Decoction of Gypsum Fibrosum and Three Yellows	(211)
Decoction of Ginseng for Nourishing Qi and Ying	(212)
Ease Powder	(214)
Decoction of Aneglicae Pubescentis and Taxilli	(216)
Decoction for Pus Drainage and Relieving Pain	(218)
Xiaojin Pellet	(219)
Decoction for Warming Yang	(220)
Decoction of Persicae for Purgation	(222)
Major Decoction for Purging Down Digestive Qi	(223)
Major Decoction of Bupleurum	(225)
Pill of Stephaniae Tetrandrae, Zanthoxyli, Lepidii seu Descurainiae and Rhei	(226)
Powder of Bupleuri for Dispersing the Depressed Liver-Qi	(227)
Decoction of Gentianae for Purging Liver-Fire	(228)
Pulse-Activating Powder	(229)
Decoction for Rashes Subsidence	(230)
Decoction of Restoration	(232)
Decoction for Severe Phlegm-Heat Syndrome in the Chest	(233)

Decoction for Soothing the Intestine ………………………………… (233)
Decoction of Angelicae Sinensis for Analgesic ……………………… (235)
Decoction of Angelicae Sinensis for Warming Cold Limbs ………… (236)
Decoction of Indigo Naturalis for Rashes Subsidence ……………… (237)
Decoction of Sargassum for Goiter …………………………………… (239)
Pill for Eliminating Phlegm Evil ……………………………………… (240)

Chapter One
Urinary Infection

Urinary infection is the total name of pyelonephritis, cystitis and urethritis. Its main clinical symptoms are fever, lumbago, frequent micturition, urgent urination, urodynia, etc.. According to the symptoms, urinary infection falls into two kinds: acute and chronic. Acute urinary infection refers to infection lasting for less than 6 months after the onset; and chronic more than 6 months. Most of the acute one may be cured but a small number of it will become protracted and recurrent and finally develop into chronic ones due to various causes. In the end, renal function may be fade decreased. It is belonged to the category of "stranguria" and "lumbago" in traditional Chinese medicine. . As for chronic urinary infection, it has more complex pathogenesis and different clinical manifestations. The one with remarkable symptoms due to deficiency such as edema, acraturesis and emaciation should be included in the syndromes of "edema" and "consumptive disease" in traditional Chinese medicine.

ETIOLOGY AND PATHOGENESIS

Because too much food pungent and sweet in flavor and hot and fatty in nature or too much drink is taken in, damp-heat is led to flow downward into the urinary bladder; because the low orifices are unclean, dirty and turbid pathogens seize the opportunity to invade the urinary bladder so that damp-heat is formed; because damp-heat is accumulated in the lower-jiao, the qi of the urinary bladder fails to perform its function normally. In this case, there will appear urgent urination, frequent micturition and urodynia. If the disease is protected, both the spleen and kidney will become weakened, and in turn, syndromes due to both deficiency and excess will be brought about.

Urinary Infection

MAIN SYMPTOMS AND SIGNS

1. Lower tract involvement

Burning pain on urination, often with turbid, foul-smelling, or dark urine, frequency, and suprapubic or lower abdominal discomfort. There are usually no positive physical findings unless the upper tract is involved too.

Microscopic examination of a properly collected urine specimen usually shows significant bacteriuria and pyuria and occasionally hematuria. Bacteriuria is confirmed by culture. Leukocytosis is rare unless the upper tract is also involved.

2. Acute pyelonephritis

Sudden rise of body temperature to 102 to 105°F, shaking chills, aching pain in one or both costovertebral areas or flanks, and symptoms of bladder inflammation. Physical examination reveals tenderness in the region of one or both kidneys; at times, a tender kidney may be detected by palpation. Laboratory tests show polymorphonuclear leukocytosis, and the urine is laden with leukocytes. Stain of the sediment reveals numerous bacteria, usually gram-negative bacilli, and culture confirms this. In a small proportion of cases, culture is also positive.

MAIN POINTS OF DIAGNOSIS

1. Clinical manifestations are characterized by symptoms of infection such as fever, vomiting, diarrhea, pallor and loss of appetite. In infants, jaundice may be present.

2. The typical symptoms of urinary infection may include urodynia, urgency and frequency of urination, dysuria, dripping urine, pain in the lumbar region, occasionally with transient hematuria and enuresis. Infants may have irritated cry when urinating and obstinate diaper rash which are liable to be accompanied with inflammation of mucous membrane of the external genital organs.

3. Chronic recurrent infection may be accompanied with intermittent fever, lumbar soreness, fatigue and anemia, or with renal failure in severe cases.

4. In laboratory examinations, urinary sediment after centrifugation usually shows white cells and casts. In urine culture, bacterial colony counts over 100,

000/ml may permit a tentative diagnosis of urinary infection.

5. Ultrasonography of kidney, and nephropyelography may help to find the causes of urinary infection, such as deformity of urinary tract, kidney stone, obstruction, backflow of urine and hydronephrosis.

DIFFERENTIATION AND TREATMENT OF COMMON SYNDROMES

1. Damp-heat in the urinary bladder

Main Symptoms and Signs: Aversion to cold, fever, marked by persistent fever after sweating, urgent and frequent micturition, dripping discharge of urine with burning sensation and stabbing pain, nausea, vomiting, distending pain in the lower abdomen, restlessness with frequent crying in infants, urgency of urination with dark urine, red tongue with yellow or white and greasy fur, and rapid pulse.

Therapeutic Principles: Clearing away and purging pathogenic heat-fire, and inducing diuresis to treat strangury.

Recipe: *Modified Eight Health - Restoring Powder*

Herba Polygoni Avicularis	9 g
Herba Dianthi	9 g
Caulis Clematidis Armandii	3 g
Semen Plantaginis	9 g
Fructus Gardeniae	9 g
Talcum	12 g
Radix Glycyrrhizae	3 g
Herba Lophatheri	9 g
Flos Lonicerae	15 g
Rhizoma Imperatae	15 g

All the above drugs are to be decocted in water for oral administration.

Recipe: *Shiwei tongling fang*

Folium Pyrrosiae	30 g
Herba Polygoni Avicularis	12 g
Herba Dianthi	9 g

Radix et Rhizoma Rhei	6 g
Herba Lophatheri	9 g
Rhizoma Imperatae	30 g
Semen Plantaginis	15 g
Talcum	30 g
Herba Leonuri	15 g
Radix Glycyrrhizae	3 g

Administration: All the above drugs are to be decocted in water for oral administration. One dose daily.

Modification: In case of more severe chills and fever, bitter taste, nausea and vomiting, the drugs added are *Radix Bupleuri* 15 g, *Rhizoma Pinelliae* 9 g, *Radix Scutellariae* 12 g.

In the number of pus cells fails to be reduced and the tongue coating is yellow and greasy, the drugs added are *Herba Taraxaci* 30 g, *Rhizoma Smilacis Glabrae* 12 g. In case of hematuria, the drugs added are *Herba Cirii* 30 g, *Radix Rehmanniae* 30 g and *Nodus Nelumbinis Rhizomatis* 12 g.

Recipe: *Simple Prescription* 1

Herba Taraxaci	60 g

The above drug is to be decocted in water for oral administration.

Recipe: *Simple Prescription* 2

Radix Pyrrosiae	120 g

Cleaned, pounded and then decocted in water to get thick decoction for oral use.

Recipe: *Proven Prescription* 1

Herba Violae	60 g
Semen Plantaginis	60 g

All the above drugs are to be decocted in water for oral administration.

Recipe: *Proven Prescription* 2

Flos Lonicerae	30 g

Herba Lonicerae	30 g
Rhizoma Imperatae	30 g
Herba Plantaginis	30 g
Herba Lophatheri	12 g

All the above drugs are to be decocted in water for oral administration.

2. Stagnated heat in the liver and gallbladder

Main Symptoms and Signs: Fever, aversion to cold, bitter taste in the mouth, anorexia or vomiting, restlessness, frequent and precipitant urination with scanty dark urine, difficulty and pain in micturition, yellow and greasy fur of the tongue, taut and rapid pulse.

Therapeutic Principles: Purging pathogenic fire and toxin, removing pathogenic heat from the liver and gallbladder.

Recipe: *Modified Decoction of Gantian for Purging Liver — fire*

Fructus Gardeniae	9 g
Radix Scutellariae	9 g
Radix Bupleuri	9 g
Radix Rehmanniae	9 g
Semen Plantaginis	9 g
(wrapped in a piece of cloth before decoction)	
Rhizoma Alismatis	9 g
Caulis Clematidis Armandii	3 g
Cortex Phellodendri	9 g
Rhizoma Imperatae	15 g
Rhizoma Smilacis Glabrae	9 g
Radix Glycyrrhizae	3 g

All the above drugs are to be decocted in water for oral administration.

3. Deficiency of both the spleen and the kidney

Main Symptoms and Signs: Difficulty and pain in micturition and dripping urination, short breath, disinclination to speak, pale complexion, anorexia and abdominal distention, loose stool, sore waist, fatigue, weakness, pale tongue with thin and white fur, and deep, thready and weak pulse.

Therapeutic Principles: Strengthening the spleen and tonifying the kidney to eliminate dampness.

Recipe: *Modified Decoction of Four Noble Drugs* combined with *Life Preserving Pill for Replenishing the Kidney qi*

Radix Codonopsis Pilosulae	9 g
Poria	9 g
Rhizoma Atractylodis Macrocephalae	9 g
Rhizoma Dioscoreae	9 g
Fructus Corni	9 g
Semen Plantaginis (wrapped in a piece of cloth before it is to be decocted)	9 g
Rhizoma Achyranthis Bidentatae	9 g
Semen Coicis	12 g

All the above drugs are to be decocted in water for oral administration.

Modification: For those with sore waist, add 9 grams of *Ramulus Loranthi*; in case of edema, add 15 grams of *Exocarpium Benincase* and 9 grams of *Rhizoma Alismatis*.

Recipe: *Wubi shanyao wan*

Rhizoma Dioscoreae	12 g
Poria	12 g
Rhizoma Alismatis	15 g
Radix Rehmanniae Praeparata	15 g
Fructus Corni	9 g
Radix Morindae Officinalis	12 g
Semen Cuscutae	15 g
Cortex Eucommiae	12 g
Rhizoma Achyranthis Bidentatae	12 g
Fructus Schisandrae	9 g
Herba Cistanchis	12 g
Halloysitum Rubrum	6 g

Administration: All the above drugs are to be decocted in water for oral administration. One dose daily.

4. Type of retention of damp – heat due to insufficiency of the kidney – yin

Main Symptoms and Signs: Dizziness, tinnitus, soreness and weakness of the loins and knees, dry throat and lips, low fever, mild or severe frequent and urgent urination and urodynia, reddish tongue with thin coating, and taut thready rapid pulse.

Therapeutic Principles: Nourishing yin, invigorating the kidney, clearing away heat and descending fire.

Recipe: *Zhibai dihuang tang jiajian*

Radix Rehmanniae	15 g
Rhizoma Dioscoreae	10 g
Fructus Corni	9 g
Cortex Moutan	12 g
Poria	9 g
Rhizoma Alismatis	15 g
Rhizoma Anemarrhenae	12 g
Cortex Phellodendri	9 g
Herba Pyrrosiae	15 g
Herba Lophatheri	9 g

Administration:

All the above drugs are to be decocted in water for oral use. One dose daily.

5. Fire hyperactivity due to yin deficiency

Main Symptoms and Signs: Prolonged duration, difficult urination with incomplete sensation, slight distention in the lower abdomen, palpitation, shortness of breath, dry mouth and tongue, restlessness, warm sensation in the heart, palms and soles, insomnia, dreaminess. Red tongue with scanty coating, thready and rapid pulse.

Therapeutic Principles: Clear away heat and nourish yin the harmonize the heart and kidney.

Recipe:

Radix Scutellariae	9 g
Cortex Lycii	9 g
Poria	12 g
Semen Plantaginis	

(wrapped in a piece of cloth before it is to be decocted) 9 g
Radix Ophiopogonis   12 g
Lophatheri   9 g
Radix Rehmanniae   15 g
Talcum   15 g
Radix Glycyrrhizae   6 g

6. Heat – strangury

Main Symptoms and Signs: Oscillations between chills and fever, distention and pain of the hypogastrium, difficulty of urination, dark urine, burning pain of the urethra on micturition, rapid pulse and yellow coating of the tongue.

Therapeutic Principles: Dissipate heat and detoxify the body.

Recipe: *Xiao chaihu tang* and *Bazhen san jiajian*

Radix Bupleuri   30 g
Radix Scutellariae   12 g
Gypsum   40 g
Herba Polygoni Avicularis   30 g
Herba Dianthi   30 g
Polyporus   15 g
Semen Plantaginis   30 g
Talcum   18 g
Herba Taraxaci   30 g
Herba Violae   30 g
Cortex Phellodendri   10 g
Herba Lophatheri   10 g
Rhizoma Alismatis   12 g

All the above drugs are to be decocted in water for oral administration.

7. Blood – strangury

Main Symptoms and Signs: Hematuria with urethral pains and distention and pain of the hypogastrium, usually the patients with rapid pulse and yellow coating of the tongue.

Therapeutic Principles: Cool blood and detoxify the body.

Recipe: *Xiaoji yinzi jiajian*

Herba Cephalanoploris	15 g
Nodus Nelumbinis Rhizomatis	9 g
Talcum	18 g
Pollen Typhae	9 g
Radix Rehmanniae	30 g
Herba Lophatheri	9 g
Cacumen Platycladi Orientalis	12 g
Herba Violae	30 g
Herba Taraxaci	30 g
Radix Sanguisorbae	30 g
Radix Scutellariae	15 g
Flos Lonicerae	30 g
Cortex Phellodendri	15 g

All the above drugs are to be decocted in water for oral administration.

8. Consumptive-strangury

Main Symptoms and Signs: One of the strangury symptom complexes, which is chronic with exacerbation of symptoms after overwork. It is mainly manifested by dribbling of urine, vague pain of the genitalia after micturition, lassitude, lower backache, hot palms and soles, and refractory to treatment. When chronic, the patients have weak pulse, enlarged, swollen tongue with glossy coating.

Therapeutic Principles: Nourish the kidney and clear the heat.

Recipe: *Zhibai dihuang tang jiajian*

Rhizoma Anemarrhenae	12 g
Cortex Phellodendri	12 g
Radix Rehmanniae Praeparata	12 g
Rhizoma Dioscoreae	24 g
Fructus Corni	24 g
Poria	30 g
Rhizoma Alismatis	15 g
Cortex Moutan Radicis	12 g
Herba Taraxaci	30 g
Herba Violae	30 g
Ramulus Loranthi	30 g

Urinary Infection

Radix Phlomis	15 g

All the above drugs are to be decocted in water for oral administration.

Acupuncture and Moxibustion

Main points: **Pángguāngshū(BL28)**, **Zhōngjí(RN3)**, **Yīnlíngquán(SP9)** and **Tàixī(KI3)**

Compl ementary points: Add **Cìliáo(BL32)** and **Qūquán(LR8)** for damp - heat in the lower energizer; add **Shènshū(BL23)** for fire hyperactivity due to yin deficiency.

Method: The filiform needles are used. **Tàixī(KI3)** and **Shènshū(BL23)** are punctured with tonification. The other points are punctured with sedation, and the needles are retained for 15 minutes.

Medicated Diet

1. Put *mung bean* 15 g, *red bean* 15 g, *balck soybean* 15 g and *licorice powder* 9 g in the pot and boil them in water. Eat the beans and drink the soup after the beans are thoroughly done.

2. Decoct *dandelion herb* 50 g (or 100 g of fresh) into the decoction and take out the dregs. Then add *coix seed* 30 g to cook gruel and add proportional amount of *crystal sugar* to take at one draught.

4. Mung bean gruel

Semen Phaseoli Radiati	50 g
Medulla Tetrapanacis	10 g
Fructus Tritici	50 g

Process: First decoct the *ricepaper pith* in 2,000 ml of water and sift out 1,000 ml of the decoction; then make gruel with the 1,000 ml of decoction and *mung bean* and *wheat* for eating.

Directions: To be taken before meals. It can be used to treat urinary infection of the type of insufficiency of both the spleen and the kidney with retention of toxic material in the lower - jiao.

5. Tale gruel

Talcum	20 to 30 g

Herba Dianthi   10 g
Semen Oryzae Sativae   50 to 100 g

Process: First decoct the first two ingredients in an earthenware pot and remove the drugs, and then add the rice to the decoction and make gruel with them.

Directions: This recipe can be widely used to treat acute urinary tract infection manifested as all the types. Pregnant women should avoid it.

It also can be chosen to treat urinary infection manifested as the type of damp-heat of the lower-jiao with retention of toxic material in the urinary bladder.

Prevention

1. Keep the progenital area clean, change undershorts regularly and pay attention to menstrual and gravidic hygiene.

2. Treat focal purulent disease change timely to avoid hematogenous spread and take the important measure of removing the inducing factors such as urinary obstruction.

Chapter Two
Mammary Development

When one side or both sides of the male breast undergo a gynecogenic development or hypermastia, this disorder of mammary development is equal to Rǔlì (puberty mastitis) in traditional Chinese medicine. If its onset is in the adolescence, it is called adolescent (primary) disorder of mammary development, which is common in young children of about 10. If its onset is in those after middle age, it is called male (secondary) disorder of mammary development (Gynecomastia).

ETIOLOGY AND PATHOGENESIS

The nipple is connected with the liver, the breast of a female with the stomach, the breast of a male with the kidney. Disorder of qi is the main cause in male, while disorder of blood in female.

Emotional disorder and anger impair the liver, leading to stagnation of the liver - qi. Stagnation of the liver - qi results in production of fire. The fire turns body fluid into phlegm. The phlegm and the stagnated qi unite as one, causing this disease.

Fire due to stagnation of the liver - qi goes down to burn the kidney = yin. Or, over sexual intercourse impairs the kidney, leading to insufficiency of the kidney - yin and flaring - up of fire of deficiency type. The fire burns body fluid into phlegm. The fire and the phlegm get together to cause this disease.

Weak spleen and stomach in adolescent female will dysfunction in transportation and transformation, which reduces the supplement of qi and blood, leads to dysfunction of Chong and Ren Channels, results in incoordination between qi and blood and causes stagnation of blood in the vessels, with this disease coming into being.

Insufficiency of the kidney - essence and blood in adolescent male makes the liver fail to be nourished, which leads to stagnation of the liver - qi and accumulation of phlegm and causes this disease.

MAIN SYMPTOMS AND SIGNS

Oval middle - hard distinctly - bordered smooth movable mildly - tender or distending - painful masses at the center of the areola of one or both breasts, not enlarged axillary lymph nodes, no general symptoms in adolescent disorder of mammary development, male disorder of mammary development with the above symptoms and hypermastia (looking like breasts of developed female), chocking sensation in the chest, anxiety, irritability, or soreness and weakness of the loins and knees, dizziness, vertigo, sexual hypesthesia, sharp voice, and reduced beard. If the disorder is limited in one breast and the mass is harder, differentiation from mammary cancer is needed.

MAIN POINTS OF DIAGNOSIS

1. **Adolescent disorder of mammary development:** The breasts may be enlarged bilaterally or unilaterally in their adolescence. Mastoplasia occurs under the areola of mamma. It is associated with tenderness which may last for about half a year and then disappear.

2. **Gynecomastia:** When it occurs in old patients, they are mostly above the age of 50. There will be some limited lumps which are palpable under the areola of mamma. They are hard and tenacious, well limited, smooth and there is no adhesion between them and the skin or deep tissues.

3. The patient is usually associated with diseases of hypoplasia of sex glands, such as cryptorchism, secondary testitis, traumatic atrophy of testis(es), orchioncus, etc..

4. Those who are suffering from cirrhosis sometimes may have mammary development due to the disturbance of their intermediate metabolism of steroid hormone.

5. If the patient has been using medicine such as estrin, isoniazid and chlorpromazine for a long time, mastauxe will be possible.

DIFFERENTIATION AND TREATMENT OF COMMON SYNDROMES

External Treatment

If there are distinct distention in the breast and obvious tenderness on the lumps, take 20 grams of *Natrii Sulphas* and dissolve it in 10 ml of boiling water for wet dressing which is to be applied onto the affected part or use *Paste for Activating Yang and Resolving Coagulation of Yin*, combined with *Hituixiao Powder*, which is placed onto the same part. Generally, the dressing should be changed every seven days.

Operative Therapy

If the breast is too large and has distending pain or anxiety caused by the trouble occurs or there is no result after pharmacotherapy or it is suspected of mammary cancer, an operation should be carried out.

Internal Treatment

1) The type of deficiency of the kidney – yin

Main Symptoms and Signs: In addition to mastauxe it is often associated with dizziness, tinnitus, aching in the waist and knees, dryness of the throat and mouth, red tongue and the thready and rapid pulse.

Therapeutic Principles: Nourishing the kidney – yin by removing phlegm to resolve masses.

Recipe: *Zuogui wan jiajian*

Radix Rehmanniae Praeparata	24 g
Rhizoma Dioscoreae	12 g
Fructus Corni	12 g
Semen Cuscutae	12 g
Fructus Lycii	12 g
Colla Cornus Cervi	12 g
Colla Plastri Testudinis	12 g

Fructus Trichosanthis	12 g
Bulbus Fritillariae	10 g
Rhizoma Pinelliae	10 g

All the above drugs are to be decocted in water for oral administration.

2) **The type of deficiency of the kidney − yang**

Main Symptoms and Signs: Besides mastauxe, the disease is often associated with aversion to cold, ache and weakness of the lumbus and knees, sexual impotence and loose stool, thin and whitish fur on the tongue and deep and thready pulse.

Therapeutic Principles: Warming and nourishing the kidney − yang with removing phlegm to resolve masses.

Recipe: *Yougui wan jiajian*

Radix Rehmanniae Praeparata	24 g
Rhizoma Dioscoreae	12 g
Semen Cuscutae	12 g
Fructus Lycii	12 g
Cortex Eucommiae	12 g
Colla Cornus Cervi	12 g
Fructus Corni	9 g
Radix Aconiti Praeparata	9 g
Cortex Cinnamomi	9 g
Radix Angelicae Sinensis	9 g
Semen Sinapis Album	9 g
Bulbus Fritillariae	9 g

All the above drugs are to be decocted in water for oral administration.

3) **the type of stagnation of the liver − qi and accumulation of phlegm**

Main Symptoms and Signs: Chocking sensation in the chest, anxiety, irritability, impatience, reddish tongue with thin white coating, and thready taut pulse.

Therapeutic Principles: Soothing the liver and promoting the flow of the liver − qi, resolving phlegm and dispersing masses.

Recipe: *Ruli tang*

Radix Bupleuri	10 g

Rhizoma Cyperi	10 g
Bulbus Fritillariae Thunbergii	10 g
Pericarpium Citri Reticulatae Viride	10 g
Rhizoma Pinelliae	10 g
Folium Citri Reticulatae	10 g
Thallus Laminariae seu Echloniae	15 g
Sargassum	
Fructus Trichosanthis	15 g
Concha Ostreae	30 g
Spica Prunellae	15 g
Radix Salviae Miltiorrhizae	15 g

All the above drugs are to be decocted in water for oral administration. It is taken warm in the morning and evening, one dose daily. One course of treatment consisting of 2 weeks.

Modification: In case of harder masses, the drug added is *Squama Manitis Praeparata* 10 g. In case of fullness in the chest and pain in the hypochondriac region, the drug added is *Radix Curcumae* 10 g.

4) The type of insufficiency of the liver and kidney

Main Symptoms and Signs: Soreness and weakness of the loins and knees, dizziness, vertigo, blackened orbits, sexual hypesthesia, reddened tongue with little coating, and thready slightly rapid pulse.

Therapeutic Principles: First of all tonifying the liver and kidney and secondly resolving phlegm and softening masses.

Recipe: *Liuwei dihuang tang jiajian*

Radix Rehmanniae Praeparata	30 g
Fructus Corni	10 g
Poria	10 g
Rhizoma Alismatis	10 g
Cortex Moutan Radicis	10 g
Rhizoma Dioscoreae	10 g
Fructus Lycii	10 g
Bulbus Fritillariae Thunbergii	15 g
Sargassum	15 g
Fructus Trichosanthis	15 g

All the above drugs are to be decocted in water for oral administration. Take it warm in the morning and evening, one dose daily.

Modification: For those with sexual hypoessthesia, sharp voice and reduced beard, the drugs added are *Herba Epimedii* 30 g, *Radix Morindae Officinalis* 15 g, and *Cornu Cervi Degelatinatum* 10 g. In case of dry mouth and throat, the drugs added are *Carapax et Plastrum Testudinis* 10 g, *Rhizoma Anemarrhenae* 10 g, and *Cortex Phellodendri* 6 g.

Chinese Patent Medicines and Proved Recipes

1) Bolus for Tonifying the Kidney — qi: Take one bolus at one time, twice daily.

2) Modified Decoction of Epimedium and Curculigo

Rhizoma Curculiginis	10 g
Herba Epimedii	10 g
Radix Angelicae Sinensis	10 g
Rhizoma Anemarrhenae Praeparata	10 g
Fructus Trichosanthis	10 g
Radix Rehmanniae Praeparata	18 g

All the above drugs are to be decocted in water for oral administration.

3) For mild cases, Sanjie pian can be taken.

Chapter Three
Acute Glomerulonephritis

A*cute* glomerulonephritis is an immunoreactive disease caused by the deposition of immune complex in the glomeruli mainly after hemolytic streptococcal infection. The disease can also be caused by other organisms, or is involved as a part of the manifestations of other disease. Most patients can recover completely. A few cases may develop to chronic nephritis. This disease pertains to the category of "*fēngshǔi*"(wind edema) in traditional Chinese medicine.

ETIOLOGY AND PATHOGENESIS

Glomerulonephritis is a disease affecting both kidneys. In most cases, recovery from the acute stage is complete. However, progressive involvement may destroy renal tissue, in which case renal insufficiency results. Acute glomerulonephritis is most common in children 3 to 10 years of age. Although 5% or more of initial attacks occur in adults over age 50. By far the most common cause is an antecedent infection of the pharynx and tonsils or of the skin with group A B − *hemolytic streptococci*, certain strains of which are nephritogenic. In children under age 6, pyoderma(impetigo) is the most common antecedent; in older children, skin infection is rare. Nephritogenic strains commonly encountered include, for the skin, M type 49, 2 and 55; for pharyngitis, type 12, 1 and 4, rarely, nephritis may follow infections due to *pneumococci*, *staphylococci*, some bacilli and viruses, or, plasmodium malariae and exposure to some drugs, including penicillins, sulfonamides, phenytoin, aminosalicylic acid and aminoglycoside antibiotics. Rhus dermatitis and reactions to venom or chemical agents may be associated with renal disease clinically indistinguishable from glomerulonephritis.

The pathogenesis of the glomerular lesion has been further elucidated by the use of new immunologic techniques (immunofluorescence) and electron microscopy. A likely sequela to infection by nephritogenic strains of B − *hemolytic streptococci* is injury to the mesangial cells in the intercapillary space. The glomerulus may then become more easily damaged by antigen – antibody complexes developing from the immune response to the streptococcal infection. The **C3** component of complement is deposited in association with **IgG** (rarely **IgA** or **IgM**) or alone in a granular pattern on the epithelial side of the basement membrane and occasionally in subendothelial sites as well. Similar immune complex deposits in the glomeruli can often be demonstrated when the organ is other than streptococcal.

Gross examination of the involved kidney shows only punctate hemorrhages through the cortex. Microscopically, the primary alteration is in the glomeruli, which show proliferation and swelling of the mesangial and endothelial cells of the capillary tuft. The proliferation of capsular epithelium produces a thickened crescent about the tuft, and in the space between the capsule and the tuft there are collections of leukocytes, red cells and exudate. Edema of the interstitial tissue and cloudy swelling of the tubule epithelium are common. Immune complexes are demonstrable by means of immunofluorescence techniques. As the disease develops, the kidney may enlarge. The typical histologic findings in glomerulitis are enlarging crescents that become hyalinized and converted into scar tissue and obstruct the circulation through the glomerulus. Degenerative changes occur in the tubules, with fatty degeneration and necrosis and ultimate scarring of the nephron. Arteriolar thickening and obliteration become prominent.

Attack of exogenous wind, cold and dampness, improper diet and daily life or internal injury due to overstrain lead to dysfunction of the lung in clearing and regulating, of the spleen in transporting, of the kidney in opening and closing, of the urinary bladder in transforming qi, and of the tri – warmer in clearing water passage, and cause retention of water in the muscles and abdomen, resulting in edema.

MAIN SYMPTOMS AND SIGNS

Most patients have a fairly clear history of preceding streptococcal infection or exposure to a drug or other inciting agent. Usually the infection is a pharyngitis which has been sufficiently served to keep the patient away from school or work, but occasionally the infection lies elsewhere – for example, an otitis media, a leg ulcer, or a surgical wound. Sometimes the infection can only be demonstrated by a positive bacteriologic culture, or presumed from the finding of a raised *anti-streptomycin O titer*.

The patient has usually recovered from the initial infection when manifestations of nephritis appear, some 7 to 20 days after onset of the original infection. The most common presenting symptoms is edema, noted particularly in the face on first arising, hematuria is also a common first symptom, usually the urine has a brown color, but occasionally it is frankly blood-stained. Less commonly the patient complains of reduced urine output, or of bilateral dull loin pain, which is probably caused by stretching of the renal capsules.

It is important to note that the edema present at the onset of the disease is the result of reduced renal excretion of salt and water. In an adult of average size the presence of generalized edema implies a weight gain of at least 5 kg. At this stage patients have not lost enough protein in the urine to develop hypoalbuminemic edema (nephrotic syndrome), although this complication may develop later. Nor is there any good evidence for the earlier views that the edema of acute nephritis is caused either by increased capillary permeability or by heart failure.

Vague malaise, nausea and headache are common in acute nephritis, but fever is usual and patients do not usually feel really ill, although they are often distressed by the appearance of edema. In mild cases the patient may be quite asymptomatic; the disease may be picked up only by examining the urine of a person known to have had a recent streptococcal infection.

Physical examination usually shows generalized edema and mild hypertension of the order of 140 to 160 systolic, 90 to 11 diastolic. Very occasionally hypertension is severe with retinal hemorrhages and exudates, papilledema or hypertensive encephalopathy. Fluid retention, if marked, may lead to the signs of congestive cardiac failure with cardiac enlargement and triple rhythm, venous engorgement, hepatic distention and gross pulmonary and systemic edema.

Urine output is usually reduced, although the reduction is often not noticed by the patient. Complete suppression of urine is rare, and indications vary with severe attack of nephritis; this complication may develop within a few days of the onset, or urine output may gradually fall to nothing over several weeks. As might be expected, fluid retention is particularly severe in such cases, and unless rigid restriction of sodium and water has been instituted early. Edema and hypertension are particularly marked. Unless renal function returns rapidly, the symptoms of renal failure eventually appear with nausea and vomiting, twitching and pruritus, acidotic respiration and progressive anemia.

MAIN POINTS OF DIAGNOSIS

1. A vast majority of patients have hemolytic streptococcal infection 1 – 3 weeks prior to the onset of acute nephritis such as tonsillitis, angina, scarlet fever or purulent infection of the skin.

2. The onset is sudden. Edema, hypertension, albuminuria are the major manifestations accompanied with hematuria and cylindruria. In mild cases, only slight edema of eyelids and urinary changes may be present. In severe cases there may be heart failure, hypertensive encephalopathy or even renal failure.

3. Laboratory examination shows moderate albuminuria with erythrocytes and casts in the urine. *Serum creatinine* may rise slightly. **ESR** (erythrocyte sedimentation rate) may grow at speed and **ASO** (antistreptolysin O) may be positive. In some cases, throat swab culture may give a positive result of group A – *hemolytic streptococci*.

DIFFERENTIATION AND TREATMENT OF COMMON SYNDROMES

1. Wind edema

Main Symptoms and Signs: Sudden onset, fever and chill characterized by higher fever and slight chill, dry mouth, sore throat, scanty and deep – colored urine, facial edema at the beginning followed by edema all over the body especially of the face and head, red tongue with thin whitish fur, floating and rapid pulse.

Therapeutic Principles: Dispelling pathogenic wind, removing pathogenic heat and ventilating the lung to induce diuresis.

Recipe: *Modified Decoction for Relieving Edema*

Herba Ephedrae	6 g
Gypsum Fibrosum	30 g
Flos Lonicerae	20 g
Herba Leonuri	20 g

Rhizoma Imperatae	30 g
Herba Lophatheri	10 g
Radix Glycyrrhizae	3 g

All the above drugs are to be decocted in water for oral administration.

Modification: In addition to the above ingredients, the employment of the following drugs is necessary for accessory treatment: *Radix Scrophulariae* 12 g and *Radix Isatidis* 20 g for the case with marked sore throat; *Cortex Mori Radicis* 10 g and *Semen Lepidii seu Descurainiae* 10 g for the case suffering from cough with dyspnea; *Flos Chrysanthemi* 10 g and *Folium Mori* 10 g to treat headache; *Herba Cephalanoploris* 30 g to treat hematuria; and *Herba Plantaginis* 12 g to treat severe edema.

If the disorder is considered exterior syndrome of wind – cold manifested as fever, chill, stuffy nose and headache, aching pain in the body and limbs, facial edema, puffiness of eyelids, scanty urine, thin and white coating of the tongue, floating and tight pulse. The treatment should be aimed at relieving the exterior syndrome with drugs pungent in flavor and warm in property and ventilating the lung to induce diuresis. The preferable recipe for it is modified prescriptions of **Ephedra Decoction with Bighead Atractylodes** and **Decoction of Peel of Five Drugs**. The compositions are *Herba Ephedrae* 10 g, *Ramulus Cinnamomi* 6 g, *Semen Armeniacae Amarum* 6 g, *Rhizoma Atractylodis Macrocephalae* 10 g, *Pericarpium Citri Reticulatae* 10 g, *Pericarpium Arecae* 12 g, *Pericar Poriae* 15 g, *Rhizoma Alismatis* 12 g. All the above drugs are to be decocted in water for oral administration.

2. Heat – toxin edema

Main Symptoms and Signs: Boils and carbuncles on the skin, edema of the body and limbs, dry mouth, dysphoria, scanty and deep – colored urine, dry stool, red tongue with yellowish fur, slippery and rapid pulse.

Therapeutic Principles: Clear away pathogenic heat and toxic materials and inducing diuresis to reduce edema.

Recipe: *Modified Antiphlogistic Decoction of Five Drugs*

Flos Lonicerae	30 g
Fructus Forsythiae	15 g
Herba Taraxaci	30 g

Herba Violae	15 g
Radix et Rhizoma Rhei	6 g (decocted later)
Radix Scutellariae	10 g
Rhizoma Imperatae	30 g
Herba Plantaginis	12 g

All the above drugs are to be decocted in water for oral administration.

3. Water – dampness edema

Main Symptoms and Signs: Indistinct symptoms of exterior syndrome, facial edema, edema of the body and limbs, fatigue and bodily heaviness, distention in the stomach, anorexia, oliguria, white and greasy coating of the tongue, deep and slow pulse.

Therapeutic Principles: Invigorating the spleen for excreting dampness and activating yang to induce diuresis.

Recipe: Modified prescriptions of *Powder of Five Drugs with Poria* along with *Decoction of Peel of Five Drugs*

Ramulus Cinnamomi	10 g
Polyporus Umbellatus	10 g
Rhizoma Alismatis	10 g
Rhizoma Atractylodis Macrocephalae	10 g
Poria	12 g
Pericarpium Arecae	12 g
Pericar Poriae	15 g
Exocarpium Benincase	15 g
Herba Plantaginis	12 g

All the above drugs are to be decocted in water for oral administration.

Modification: In case of stagnation of dampness – heat manifested as edema of the whole body, bitter taste in the mouth, dry throat, fullness in the chest, distention in the abdomen, scanty dark urine, yellow and greasy coating of the tongue, smooth and rapid pulse, the treatment is aimed at clearing up pathogenic heat and dampness. The preferable recipe is modified prescriptions of *Two Wonderful Drugs Powder* and *Decoction for Diuresis*. The compositions are *Rhizoma Atractylodis* 10 g, *Cortex Phellodendri* 10 g, *Radix Stephaniae Tetrandrae* 10 g, *Polyporus Umbellatus* 10 g, *Rhizoma Alismatis* 10 g, *Pericarpium Arecae* 12 g, *Poria* 15 g, *Caulis Clematidis Armandii* 10 g, *Semen Phaseoli* 30 g,

Rhizoma Imperatae 30 g. All the above drugs are to be decocted in water for oral administration.

The symptoms *edema* can also be divided into *yang* and *yin* types in traditional Chinese medicine.

1. Yang edema

Main Symptoms and Signs: Heat manifestations caused by failure of the lungs to play a clearing and descending role. The clinical manifestations are mainly puffiness in the upper part of the body, particularly in the head and face, yellowish red skin, constipation, thirst and deep and frequent pulse.

Therapeutic Principles: Clear heat and excrete dampness.

Recipe:

Fructus Forsythiae	30 g
Herba Ephedrae	10 g
Gypsum Fibrosum	30 g
Flos Lonicerae	30 g
Semen Phaseoli	30 g
Rhizoma Alismatis	15 g
Herba Leonuri	60 g
Rhizoma Imperatae	60 g
Poria	30 g
Stigma Maydis	60 g
Cortex Mori Radicis	30 g
Herba Plantaginis	30 g

All the above drugs are to be decocted in water for oral administration. Two to four doses are prescribed.

2. Yin edema

Main Symptoms and Signs: Yin edema is due to the disturbance of the function of the spleen and kidney which cannot eliminate and regulate body water. Clinically, edema first appear at the lower limbs with pale or dusky skin, tastelessness, loose stools and deep retarded pulse.

Therapeutic Principles: Warm the yang and excrete dampness.

Recipe: *Jisheng shenqi wan jiajian*

Poria	30 g
Slceratium	15 g
Rhizoma Atractylodis Macrocephalae	30 g
Cortex Cinnamomi	15 g
Rhizoma Achyranthis Bidentatae	15 g
Semen Plantaginis	30 g
Radix Rehmanniae Praeparata	12 g
Rhizoma Dioscoreae	30 g
Fructus Corni	30 g
Rhizoma Alismatis	15 g
Herba Leonuri	60 g
Rhizoma Imperatae	60 g
Herba Lycopi	12 g
Radix Salviae Miltiorrhizae	40 g
Radix Astragali seu Hedysari	60 g

Administration: Decoction and dosage is the same as the above.

Acupuncture and Moxibustion

Points for *yang edema*: **Lièquē**(LU7), **Hégǔ**(LI4), **Piānlì**(LI6), **Yīnlíngquán**(SP9) and **Pángguāngshū**(BL28).

Points for yin edema: **Píshū**(BL20), **Shènshū**(BL23), **Qìhǎi**(RN6), **Zúsānlǐ**(ST36) and **Wěiyáng**(BL39).

Method: All the above points are prescribed for puncture and the needles are retained for 20 minutes.

Moxibustion can be applied to **Píshū**(BL20) and **Shènshū**(BL23) for yin edema, and **Shuǐfēn**(RN9) and **Qìhǎi**(RN6) for yang edema.

Simple Prescriptions

Recipe: *Baimaogen tang*

Rhizoma Imperatae	500 g

Administration: Decoct it with gentle heat in 2 bowls of water for the decoction, which is divided into 7 – 8 portions. One portion is taken each time, 7 – 8 time a day.

Recipe:

    Herba Leonuri   150 g

Administration: Decoct it in water for oral use. Take it four times a day. Once every four hours. The amount is reduced to children.

Recipe:

    Folium Pyrrosiae   15 – 30 g

Administration: Decoct it in water for drink taken instead of tea.

Medicated Diet

1. Make 3 big bowls of soup with 500 g of *waxground* and take the soup in 3 separate doses. It is applicable to the types of wind – heat accumulation in the lung and of damp – heat accumulation.

2. Stew one big carp and 60 g of *red bean* to make soup for drinking at one meal. Avoid the table salt. It is suitable for the cases with distinct dropsy, dark urine and difficult urination.

3. Decoct 120 g of *red bean* and 9 g of *pokeberry root* together with water to make decoction for drinking. Take the decoction for 3 to 5 days successively.

4. Cook 120 g of *red bean* and 250 g of *cogongrass rhizome* together with water till the water is dried. Get rid of the *cogongrass rhizome* and take the *red bean* several times by chewing well.

5. Parch 2 *dried frogs*, 7 *mole crickets* and 15 g of *bottle gourd peel* together first, and then grind them into powder or make the powder into pills. Take the powder or the pills with warm wine, 6 g each time and 3 times a day.

Prevention

1. Keep the skin clean lest it be infected.
2. Try to prevent and timely treat infection of the upper respiratory tract.
3. Try to avoid attack by cold and overstrain.

Chapter Four
Chronic Glomerulonephritis

Chronic Glomerulonephritis is an allergic disease caused by a wide variety of etiological factors. Only a small percentage of cases are obviously due to the progression of acute nephritis. The majority of patients with chronic nephritis have no history of acute nephritis. The disease is common in young adults and middle aged people. Its course is long and the prognosis is poor. In traditional Chinese medicine, this disease is categorized as "Shuǐ zhǒng" (edema), "Xū láo" (consumptive diseases), "Yāo tòng" (lumbago), etc..

ETIOLOGY AND PATHOGENESIS

Attack of exopathogens, weakness of the spleen and kidney, and disturbance in both distribution of body fluid and in functioning of Qi lead to edema. Long-term edema results in insufficiency of the liver, spleen and kidney, weakness of the spleen in the function of transportation and transformation, inability of the kidney to separate the clear from the turbid, and gradual failure of the whole body to perform its qi function. In this case, symptoms due to weakened body resistance and prevailing pathogens will result.

MAIN POINTS OF DIAGNOSIS

There are three types of chronic nephritis according to the clinical features.

1. **Common type:** The course of this type is persistent. The quantitative examination of urinary protein is at a range between 1.5 g and 3.5 g per day. Patients may have hypertension, hematuria, cylindruria and decrease of renal function.

2. **Nephrotic type:** In addition to the features of the common type, quantitative examination of urinary protein is greater than 3.5 g per day, the serum albu-

min is less than 3.5 g percent. Marked edema is the characteristic feature of this type.

3. **Hypertensive type**: A persistent hypertension is the predominant manifestation of this type of chronic nephritis besides the features of the common type.

DIFFERENTIATION AND TREATMENT OF COMMON SYNDROMES

1. Deficiency of the spleen – yang and kidney – yang

Main Symptoms and Signs: Pale complexion, lassitude, listlessness, aversion to cold, cold limbs, high – grade edema, abdominal distension, anorexia, soreness of the waist, oliguria, thin and whitish coating of the tongue, deep and fine pulse.

Therapeutic Principles: Warming yang of the spleen and kidney to promote diuresis.

Recipe: *Modified Decoction for Reinforcing the Spleen*

Radix Codonopsis Pilosulae	15 g
Radix Astragali seu Hedysari	15 g
Radix Aconiti Praeparata	10 g
Rhizoma Atractylodis Macrocephalae	15 g
Poria	15 g
Cortex Cinnamomi	6 g
Pericarpium Arecae	12 g
Rhizoma Alismatis	15 g
Semen Plantaginis	30 g

(wrapped in a piece of cloth before decoction)

All the above drugs are to be decocted in water for oral administration.

Modification: If the edema is mild but persistent, it reveals the deficiency of spleen – qi, the treatment should be aimed at replenishing qi and invigorating the spleen to induce diuresis. *Modified tetrandra and astragalus decoction* is preferred for the treatment. The compositions are: *Radix Stephaniae Tetrandrae* 10 g, *Radix Astragali seu Hedysari* 15 g, *Rhizoma Atractylodis Macrocephalae* 15 g, *Radix Codonopsis Pilosulae* 15 g, *Poria* 15 g, *Polyporus Umbellatus* 12 g, *Rhizoma Alismatis* 12 g, *Pericarpium Citri Reticulatae* 10 g, *Radix Gly-*

cyrrhizae 3 g. All the above drugs are to be decocted in water for oral administration.

Recipe: *Shipi yin*

Radix Aconiti Lateralis Praeparata	9 g
Rhizoma Zingiberis Recens	6 g
Fructus Tsaoko	9 g
Poria	15 g
Rhizoma Atractylodis Macrocephalae	12 g
Fructus Chaenomelis	9 g
Pericarpium Arecae	9 g
Cortex Magnoliae Officinalis	9 g
Radix Aucklandiae	9 g
Radix Glycyrrhizae	6 g
Fructus Jujubae	5 dates
Rhizoma Zingiberis Recens	3 slices

All the above drugs are to be decocted in water for oral administration.

Modification: In case of shortness of breath, acratia and severe deficiency of qi, the drugs added are *Radix Ginseng* 6 – 9 g, *Radix Astragali seu Hedysari* 15 g.

In case of severe edema, the drugs added are *Rhizoma Alismatis* 30 g, *Semen Phaseoli* 30 g and *Semen Plantaginis* 30 g.

Recipe: *Jisheng shenqi wan* and *Zhenwu tang*

Radix Rehmanniae	15 g
Rhizoma Dioscoreae	12 g
Fructus Corni	9 g
Poria	15 g
Rhizoma Alismatis	15 g
Cortex Moutan	9 g
Rhizoma Achyranthis Bidentatae	9 g
Semen Plantaginis (decocted after being wrapped in a piece of cloth)	9 g
Radix Aconiti Lateralis Praeparata	12 g
Rhizoma Atractylodis Macrocephalae	12 g
Radix Paeoniae Alba	9 g

Rhizoma Zingiberis Recens	3 g
Radix Glycyrrhizae	3 g

All the above drugs are to be decocted in water for oral administration.

Modification: For palpitation and dark purple lips, the drugs added are *Ramulus Cinnamomi* 9 - 12 g,

Radix Salviae Miltiorrhizae 15 - 30 g.

For dyspnea and sweating, the drugs added are *Radix Ginseng* 6 - 9 g, *Gecko* 12 g.

2. Hyperactivity of Yang due to Deficiency of Yin

Main Symptoms and Signs: Indistinct edema, headache, dizziness, tinnitus, dry mouth, irritability, feverish sensation in the palms and soles, palpitation, insomnia, red tongue, taut and thready pulse.

Therapeutic Principles: Nourishing yin and suppressing hyperactive yang.

Recipe: *Bolus of Six Drugs Including Rehmannia and Adding Wolfberry and Chrysanthemum with additional ingredients*

Fructus Lycii	15 g
Flos Chrysanthemi	10 g
Radix Rehmanniae	15 g
Radix Rehmanniae Praeparata	15 g
Fructus Corni	12 g
Cortex Moutan Radicis	10 g
Rhizoma Dioscoreae	15 g
Poria	12 g
Rhizoma Alismatis	10 g
Plastrum Testudinis	15 g
Ramulus Uncariae cum Uncis	20 g
Cortex Eucommiae	10 g
Concha Haliotidis	30 g

All the above drugs are to be decocted in water for oral administration.

3. Retention of Damp - heat in the Body

Main Symptoms and Signs: Flushed face, obesity, edema, distention of head, headache, dry mouth, irritability, constipation, prolonged hormonotherapy, thin and yellowish or yellowish and greasy coating of the tongue, taut and rapid or slippery and rapid pulse.

Therapeutic Principles: Clearing away pathogenic heat and dampness.

Recipe: *Modified Decoction of Gentian for Purging Liver − fire*

Radix Gentianae	10 g
Radix Scutellariae	10 g
Fructus Gardeniae	10 g
Caulis Clematidis Armandii	10 g
Rhizoma Alismatis	10 g
Semen Plantaginis	12 g
(wrapped in a piece of cloth during decocting)	
Radix Rehmanniae	12 g
Cortex Phellodendri	10 g
Herba Taraxaci	20 g
Rhizoma Imperatae	30 g

All the above drugs are to be decocted in water for oral administration.

4. Type of Deficiency of Both the Spleen and Kidney and Insufficiency of Qi and Blood

Main Symptoms and Signs: Pale complexion, acratia of the limbs, general edema, fatigue, less sleep, poor appetite, dizziness, tinnitus, soreness and weakness of the loins and knees, pale tongue with thin white coating, and deep weak pulse.

Therapeutic Principles: Strengthening the spleen, benefiting the kidney and tonifying both qi and blood.

Recipe: *Dabuyuan jian* and *Guipi tang*

Radix Codonopsis	15 g
Radix Astragali seu Hedysari	15 g
Rhizoma Atractylodis Macrocephalae	10 g
Poria	
Fructus Lycii	15 g
Radix Angelicae Sinensis	15 g
Radix Rehmanniae Praeparata	15 g
Cortex Eucommiae	12 g

Arillus Longan	9 g
Radix Aucklandiae	6 g
Radix Glycyrrhizae	6 g
Fructus Jujubae	5 dates

Modification: For poor appetite and abdominal distention, the drugs added are *Fructus Hordei Germinatus* 12 g, *Fructus Crataegi* 12 g, *Massa Medicata Fermentata* 12 g, *Pericarpium Citri Reticulatae* 6 g, *Fructus Amomi* 6 g.

5. Deficiency of the Spleen and Kidney and Upward-going of Turbid Yin

Main Symptoms and Signs: Dim complexion with edema, listlessness, emaciation, choking and distending sensation in the chest and abdomen, anorexia, nausea, vomiting, even urinary odor in the mouth, diarrhea or constipation, oliguria, palpitation, shortness of breath, even restlessness, coma, convulsion, pale and enlarged tongue with white greasy or grayish yellow and greasy coating, and deep thready or taut thready pulse.

Therapeutic Principles: Strengthening body resistance, detoxicating and descending the turbid.

Recipe: *Wenpi tang*

Radix Aconiti Lateralis Praeparata	12 g
Radix Ginseng	10 g
Rhizoma Zingiberis Recens	6 g
Radix et Rhizoma Rhei	5–10 g
Rhizoma Pinelliae	10 g
Pericarpium Citri Reticulatae	9 g
Poria	12 g
Rhizoma Atractylodis Macrocephalae	9 g
Radix Glycyrrhizae	6 g

Modification: For fever, dysphoria and yellow greasy tongue coating, the drugs added are *Rhizoma Corydalis* 9 g, *Fructus Gardeniae* 9 g.

For convulsion, the drug added is *Concha Ostreae* 30 g.

6. Treatment of Several Main Symptoms

1) Proteinuria

(1) For proteinuria with fever, sore throat and yellow tongue coating

Recipe:

Flos Lonicerae	30 g
Fructus Forsythiae	15 g
Rhizoma Cimicifugae	9 g
Periostracum Cicadae	9 g
Herba Hedyotis Diffusae	15 g
Folium Pyrrosiae	30 g
Rhizoma Imperatae	30 g
Herba Lophatheri	9 g
Herba Leonuri	12 g
Radix Platycodi	9 g
Rhizoma Belamcandae	9 g
Radix Scutellariae	15 g
Radix Glycyrrhizae	6 g

All the above drugs are to be decocted in water for oral administration.

(2) For proteinuria with symptoms of deficiency of the spleen and kidney and pale tongue with white coating

Recipe:

Fructus Lycii	15 g
Fructus Rubi	12 g
Semen Cuscutae	15 g
Fructus Schisandrae	9 g
Semen Plantaginis (decocted after being wrapped in a piece of cloth)	
Fructuss Rosae Laevigatae	9 g
Semen Euryales	15 g
Radix Astragali seú Hedysari	15 g
Folium Pyrrosiae	15 g
Rhizoma Imperatae	30 g

All the above drugs are to be decocted in water for oral administration.

2) **High concentration urea nitrogen in blood**

(1) Treatment conducted according to what is stated in type of Deficiency of the spleen and kidney and upward-going of turbid yin

(2) Retention－edema

Recipe:

Radix et Rhizoma Rhei	9 g
Radix Sanguisorbae	30 g
Radix Aconiti Lateralis Praeparata	12 g
Concha Ostreae	60 g

Administration: Decocted in water to get 200 ml of the decoction for retention－edema, once daily.

3) 3) **Hematuria**

(1) Treatment based on what is described in **DIFFERENTIATION AND TREATMENT OF COMMON SYNDROMES**(2) Drugs considerably added are

Herba Cirii	30 g
Herba Leonuri	12 g
Rhizoma Imperatae	30 g
Radix Rehmanniae	15 g
Cortex Moutan	15 g
Nodus Nelumbinis Rhizomatis	9 g

(3) *Guipi tang*

Acupuncture and Moxibustion

Main Points: **Shuǐfēn**(RN9), **Qìhǎi**(RN6), **Shènshū**(BL23), **Píshū**(BL20), **Zúsānlǐ**(ST36), **Yīnlíngquán**(SP9), **Sānjiāoshū**(BL22), **Guānyuán**(RN4) and **Fùliū**(KI7).

Compl ementary Pointss: Add **Shuǐgōu**(DU26) for facial puffiness; add **Zúlínqì**(GB4) and **Shāngqiū**(SP5) for edema on the pedis dorsum.

Method: Use the filiform needles to puncture the points with tonification or apply moxibustion.

Medicated Diet

1. Get 1 *black carp* and cut it open. Remove its internal organs. Wrap it with mud and roast it in charcoal fire until white smoke comes out. Then take it out and grind it into powder when it gets cool. Take it with warm boiled water, 2 spoonful each time, 3 times a day. One carp makes up one dose. Salt is **prohib-**

ited. It is applicable to the patients with the deficiency of the spleen yang and kidney yang.

2. Decoct 60 g of fresh *cogongrass rhizome* (30 g if the dried is used) in water to drink frequently.

3. Parch *sesame seed* and grind it into powder. Then take it infused in boiling water added with sugar. The recipe is applicable to the patients with deficiency of the lower energizer due to protracted illness.

4. Cook a big *crucian carp* in 500 g with one *garlic bulb*, 3 g of *black pepper*, 3 g of *pricklyash peel*, 3 g of *tangerine peel*, 3 g of *amomum fruit*, 3 g of *long pepper* and 3 g of *green Chinese onion* into thick soup to take as food.

5. Make a small hole in one *egg*, put seven grains of *white pepper* into it, seal the hole with flour and wrap the egg with wet paper. Then steam it in a food steamer until it is done. The *egg* and the *pepper* are to be taken together after the egg is shelled, two eggs per day for adults, one for children, ten days making up one course of treatment. The second course of treatment is to begin following a suspension of three days. It is used to treat chronic nephritis manifested as the type of insufficiency of both the spleen and the kidney with deficiency of essence and blood.

6. Thick Crucian Carp Soup

Carassius Auratus	500 g
Bulbus Allii	one
Fructus Piperis Nigri	3 g
Pericarpium Citri Reticulatae	3 g
Pericarpium Zanthoxyli	3 g
Fructus Amomi	3 g
Fructuss Piperis Longi	3 g
Bulbus Allii Fistulosi	
thick sauce made from soybean	
table salt	

Put all the other ingredients into the belly of the fish, and cook it; then make thick soup with it. It is to be taken after seasoned. Applicable to chronic nephritis of all types.

7. Honeyed Prepared Rhizome of Rehmannia and Chinese Yam

Radix Rehmanniae Praeparata	60 g
Rhizoma Dioscoreae	60 g

Mel   500 g

Wash the first two ingredients clean quickly, place them in an earthenware pot, pour in three big bowls of water, decoct them over slow fire for forty minutes and get a half bowl of the decoction; then add another bowl of cold water to the remaining drug, decoct them for thirty minutes until half bowl of the decoction is left and sift it out, mix the two half bowls of decoction with the honey, pour the mixture into a ceramic basin, cover it so as not to let any steam get into the basin. Finally, steam it with strong fire for two hours, and when it becomes cool, put it into a bottle and cover it tightly. It is to be taken after meals with warm boiled water, twice a day, one spoonful each time. Those who are debilitated due to chronic nephritis can take it as nourishment.

Qigong

Relax the whole body. Get rid of the distracting thoughts and raise the tongue tip against the hard palate. First knock the teeth for 36 times. Stir the saliva in the mouth with the tongue. Swallow the saliva in 3 parts and send it to **Dantian** with the mind. Then imagine a black qi. When inhaling, breathe it in through the nose and fill the whole mouth with it; when exhaling, send the black qi slowly to both kidneys and then into **Dantian**. Do it for 6 to 12 times.

Prevention

Try to prevent and treat infection of the upper respiratory tract and avoid overstrain.

Chapter Five
Nephrotic Syndrome

Nephrotic Syndrome can be caused by a wide variety of glomerular diseases. It may follow bacterial or viral infections, malignant tumors and administration of some drugs. Some immune diseases, such as systemic lupus erythematosus, allergic purpura and diabetes mellitus can be complicated by nephrotic syndrome. This disease is included in the categories of *Shuǐ zhǒng*, and *Xū láo* (consumptive diseases) in traditional Chinese medicine.

MAIN POINTS OF DIAGNOSIS

1. Heavy proteinuria, accompanied with edema and hypoproteinemia, are three major manifestations of this syndrome. Urinary protein excretion exceeds 3.5 g per day. The serum albumin is lower than 30 g per liter. Severe edema may appear if serum albumin is lower than 15 g per liter.
2. The alteration of blood pressure varies with different types of the disease. Hyperlipemia is common, particularly increased cholesterol.
3. About 75 percent of cases with nephrotic syndrome are caused by primary glomerular diseases. In children nearly 80 percent of cases are nephrotic syndrome of minute lesion type. The rest are secondary to other diseases. Renopuncture biopsy is of much help in confirming the cases of the disease and indicating treatment.

DIFFERENTIATION AND TREATMENT OF COMMON SYNDROMES

1. insufficiency of the Spleen - yang and Kidney - yang
Main Symptoms and Signs: Sallow complexion, mental fatigue, cold extremi-

ties, bodily edema which is more severe in the region below the waist, anorexia, loose stool, weakness of the loins, oliguria, pale or plump moist tongue with whitish smooth fur, deep, thready and weak pulse.

Therapeutic Principles: Warming the kidney, strengthening the spleen and inducing diuresis to alleviate edema.

Recipe: *Modified Drink for Reinforcing the Spleen* in combination with *Diuretic Decoction for Strengthening Yang of the Spleen and Kidney*

Radix Astragali seu Hedysari	30 g
Radix Codonopsis Pilosulae	15 g
Rhizoma Atractylodis Macrocephalae	15 g
Poria	15 g
Semen Coicis	15 g
Radix Aconiti Praeparata	10 g
Cortex Cinnamomi	5 g
Polyporus Umbellatus	12 g
Radix Aucklandiae	5 g
Herba Epimedii	10 g

All the above drugs are to be decocted in water for oral administration.

2. Warmness of the Kidney – qi

Main Symptoms and Signs: Pale complexion, general debility with desire for sleep, aversion to cold, pitting edema, hydrops in the scrotum or hydrothorax and ascites, frequent urination at night (with profuse proteinuria), pale, swollen and teeth-printed tongue with whitish fur, deep and slow pulse.

Therapeutic Principles: Strengthen the function of the kidney to stop proteinuria.

Recipe: *Kidney-yang-reinforcing Bolus with Additional Ingredients*

Radix Rehmanniae Praeparata	15 g
Rhizoma Dioscoreae	15 g
Fructus Corni	12 g
Fructus Lycii	12 g
Semen Cuscutae	15 g
Radix Aconiti Praeparata	10 g
Cortex Cinnamomi	5 g

Radix Astragali seu Hedysari	30 g
Radix Codonopsis Pilosulae	15 g
Semen Nelumbinis	15 g
Fructus Rosae Laevigatae	15 g
Semen Euryales	15 g
Poria	15 g
Polyporus Umbellatus	12 g

All the above drugs are to be decocted in water for oral administration.

Modification: If the case is complicated with symptoms of dampness and heat, 10 grams of *Cortex Phellodendri*, 15 grams of *Talcum* and 20 grams of *Semen Coicis* ought to be added to the recipe.

Chapter Six
Urolithiasis

Urolithiasis is the general term for *Calculi* at the different parts of the urinary system. It is a common disease and it is one of the major disorder in this system including calculus of the kidney, ureteral calculus, vesical calculus and urethral calculus. The cause of urolithiasis is very complicated, and it is considered to be closely related to the environmental factors, certain areas, affections of the whole body and the urinary system. This disease belongs to the categories of "Shālin" (strangury from urolithiasis), "Shílin" (strangury caused by urinary calculus) and "Xuèlin" (strangury complicated by hematuria) in traditional Chinese medicine.

MAIN SYMPTOMS AND SIGNS

Often a stone trapped in a calix in the renal pelvis is asymptomatic. If a stone produces obstruction in a calix or at the ureteropelvic junction, dull flank pain or even colic may occur. Hematuria and symptoms of accompanying infection may be present. Flank tenderness and abdominal distention may be the only finding. \ ; The urine may contain red cells, white cells and protein. **X - ray** examination will reveal radiation stone. Excretory and retrograde urograms help to delineate the site and degree of obstruction and to confirm the presence of nonopaque stones (uric acid).

MAIN POINTS OF DIAGNOSIS

1. Symptoms

1) Calculus of the Kidney: There is a dull pain in the lower loins of the affected side, when the stones in the kidney move, a severe pain will be produced. In the mean time, it radiates along the ureter to the lower abdomen and the perineal region which is associated with different degrees of hematuria. If the case turns

into a complicated infection, the patient may have fever and pus cells in the urine.

2) **Ureteral Calculus**: In the lumbar region there is an acute pain which is often associated with hematuria. When the stones happens to be in the upper 1/3 part of the ureter, the pain will be in the costovertebral angle region and radiate to the part above iliac crest and external side of the abdomen. When the stones descend, the region of pain will also come down with the pain radiating to the thigh, testicle or vulva region.

3) 3) **Vesical Calculus**: There is a pain in urination and the pain is often severest at the end of urination. This pain mainly occurs in the lower abdomen and may radiate to the perineum and balanus. Other symptoms are often difficulty of interruption in micturition and hematuria at the end of urination, urgent and frequent micturition.

4) **Urethral Calculus**: Pain in the urination, thready or dribbling urination, or even retention of urine may appear.

2. Signs

The patients who have kidney calculus will have a percussion pain or a tenderness on the kidney area of the affected side. When there is an obstruction caused by kidney calculus and ureteral calculus and posterior urethral calculus, stones can be felt in rectal examination. In the case of anterior urethral calculus, a hard lump with tenderness may be felt in the local region.

3. **Laboratory Examination**: Through urine test the number of red blood cells is often found increased. When the function of kidney is suspected of being impaired, urea nitrogen and creatinine tests will be necessary.

4. **X-ray Examination**: The urogram will show the majority of the stones. Use excretion urography or retrograde urography to help you find out the positions of the stones and the functions of both kidneys.

5. Cystoscopy, "B" type ultrasonography and isotope renogram will be helpful for clinical diagnosis.

DIFFERENTIATION AND TREATMENT OF COMMON SYNDROMES

The following therapies are good for those cases in which the transverse diameter of the stones in the kidney and ureter is less than 1 cm; the transverse diameter of the stones the urinary bladder is less than 2 cm and there is no serious obstruction and infection, and the function of kidney is in a good condition.

Traditional Chinese medicine and Chinese herbal drugs are of definite and unique curative effects in treating urolithiasis. In clinical practice, in addition to differentiation of its characteristics, it is necessary to examine the deficiency or the excess of the syndrome as well as its transformation. It is also necessary to combine differentiation of symptoms and signs with differentiation of diseases, to select emphatically drugs possessing the property of expelling or dissolving stones in the use of "purging" method. It is absolutely inappropriate to expel the stones blindly. Though the vibrating wave lithotripsy which is commonly used at present may achieve an ideal effect, yet its lithontriptic action on renal calculi is evidently poorer than on ureter calculi. In part of the patients, though the stones are broken into pieces, yet they are not to be expelled or thoroughly expelled. Therefore the use of Chinese herbal drugs as adjuvants is quite necessary. Besides, the question of stone re-occurrence is far from being solved. But in the practice of traditional Chinese medicine, when the stones are expelled, on the basis of symptom-sign differentiation, the methods of strengthening spleen to osmose damp, regulating qi to eliminate stagnancy, expelling wind to dissolve calculi, draining water to open ureter and benefiting qi to strengthen kidney can be adopted, so that these methods can be regarded as the effective means in prevention and medication.

1. Internal Treatment

1) Qi-stagnation type

Main Symptoms and Signs: There is distending pain, dull ache or even paroxysmal colicky pain in the waist and the lower abdomen, accompanied with nausea, vomiting and hematuria, tongue with white and greasy fur and tight and taut pulse.

Therapeutic Principles: Promoting the circulation of qi, inducing diuresis, relieving strangury and removing the stones.

Recipe: *Modified Pyrrosia Decoction*

Herba Lysimachiae	30 g
Folium Pyrrosiae	15 g
Herba Dianthi	15 g
Semen Plantaginis	15 g
(to be wrapped in a piece of cloth before decoction)	
Fructus Malvae Verticillatae	15 g
Talcum	15 g
Rhizoma Alismatis	15 g
Fructus Aurantii	15 g
Semen Vaccariae	15 g
Semen Raphani	15 g
Caulis Aristolochiae Manshuriensis	6 g
Radix et Rhizoma Rhei	3 – 6 g

All the above drugs are to be decocted in water for oral administration.

Recipe:

Herba Lysimachiae	30 g
Spora Lygodii	15 g
Folium Pyrrosiae	12 g
Semen Vaccariae	12 g
Rhizoma Sparganii	9 g
Rhizoma Zedoariae	9 g
Squama Manitis	9 g
Fructus Aurantii	9 g
Radix Linderae	9 g
Radix Cyathulae	9 g
Cortex Magnoliae Officinalis	6 g

All the above drugs are to be decocted in water for oral administration.

2) **Damp – heat type**

Main Symptoms and Signs: There is a continuous pain in the waist or the lower abdomen accompanied with fever, frequent micturition, urgent urination, urodynia, cloudy or bloody urine, and pyuria, tongue with yellow and greasy fur and slippery rapid or taut rapid pulse.

Therapeutic Principles: Clearing away pathogenic heat and dampness, relieving strangury and removing the stones.

Recipe: *Modified Eight Health Restoring Powder*

Herba Lysimachiae	15 g
Herba Polygoni Avicularis	15 g
Herba Dianthi	15 g
Talcum	15 g
Cortex Phellodendri	15 g
Fructus Gardeniae	15 g

Semen Plantaginis
(to be wrapped in a piece of cloth before it is decocted in water with other drugs)

Radix et Rhizoma Rhei	12 g
Radix Glycyrrhizae	12 g

3) **Mixture of deficiency and excess**

(1) **Bias deficiency of kidney - yin**

Main Symptoms and Signs: Acute pain in loins and lower abdomen, vexatious heat and thirst, hematuria or painful urination, low fever and sweating, weak waist and knees, red tongue proper with scant fur, slender rapid pulse. They correspond to patients with urinary lithiasis complicated with chronic infection of urinary tract.

Recipe:

Herba Lysimachiae	30 g
Rhizoma Imperatae	30 g
Spora Lygodii	15 g
Radix Rehmanniae	12 g
Rhizoma Dioscoreae	12 g
Poria	12 g
Rhizoma Alismatis	12 g
Rhizoma Aremarrhenae	9 g
Cortex Phellodendri	9 g
Cortex Mori Radicis	9 g
Fructus Corni	9 g

(2) **Bias deficiency of kidney − yang**

Main Symptoms and Signs: Distention pain at loins and lower abdomen, fatigue, aversion to cold, cold limbs, long clear urination, or with occasional hematuria, frequent nocturia, light tongue proper with white fur, deep slender pulse. They correspond to patients with renal calculi, urethral calculi of lingering sick course complicated with hydronephrosis.

Recipe:

Herba Lysimachiae	30 g
Radix Astragali seu Hedysari	30 g
Spora Lygodii	15 g
Endothelium Corneum Gigeriae Galli	12 g
Folium Pyrrosiae	12 g
Semen Vaccariae	12 g
Poria	12 g
Rhizoma Atractylodis Macrocephalae	12 g
Herba Epimedii	12 g
Semen Cuscutae	12 g
Fructus Psoraleae	9 g
Fructus Aurantii	9 g

Modification: For acute abdominal pain, *Rhizoma Corydalis*, *Rhizoma Cyperi*, at 10 g each are added. For evident hematuria, *Herba Cephalanoploris*, *Radix Astragali seu Hedysari*, at 10 g each are added, *Pulvis Succinium* 5 g (to be swallowed separately). For constipation, *Radix et Rhizoma Rhei* 10 g is added. For hydronephrosis, *Semen Trigonellae*, *Herba Verbenae*, at 10 g each are added.

Administration: Drugs are decocted with water. The decoction be taken at one dose a day in three portions. A course of treatment consisting of thirty days. The second course may start after a break of a week. In the period of treatment, patients are advised to drink plenty of water and to ascend the ladder, or to do some exercises such as jumping.

63 cases of urinary lithiasis were treated with the above mentioned therapies. Of them, 45 cases were cured, 6 improved, with a total effective rate of 80.9%. The longest duration for excretion of stone was 107 days, the shortest duration 9 days, at an average of 47.8 days.

2. General Attack Therapy(GAT)

Removing the stones by general attack therapy is a comprehensive treatment consisting of a number of methods used within a short period of time with both Western medicine and Traditional Chinese medicine. It is to give full play to the therapeutic functions during the treatment so as to remove stones from the human body.

This therapy is good for those who have ureterolith with stones of less than 1 cm in diameter and have no serious infection in the urinary system, no obvious urinary tract stricture or obstruction, no or slightly hydronephrosis with the renal function in the normal range.

General Attack Scheme

Time	Measures
6:00 a.m.	Drink 500 ml of water (tea better)
6:30 a.m.	Take 50 – 75 mg of dihydrochlorothazide
7:30 a.m.	Drink 500 ml of water
8:00 a.m.	Take one dose of Chinese drug (to be decocted in water to from 200 ml of decoction)
9:30 a.m.	Use 0.5 mg of atropine or also take 10 mg of furosemide at the same time
9:40 a.m.	Electrotherapy Acupoints: connect cathode to Shènshū(**BL23**) and connect anode to Pángguāngshū(**BL28**). It is good for those who have pyelolithiasis and stones in the upper middle part of the ureter; while connect cathode to Shènshū(**BL23**) and connect anode to Shuǐdào(**ST28**). It is used for those who have stones in the lower part of the ureter; connecting cathode to Guānyuán(**RN4**) and connecting anode to Sānyīnjiāo(**SP6**) are used to treat those who have cystolith or urethral calculus. Use weak stimulation at the beginning and strong stimulation later. The needling lasts for 20 minutes.
10:00 a.m.	Get up and do exercise or some jumping.

Clinical Observation: During the process of the general attack therapy, a very careful clinical observation is required. If the painful part descends, that means the stones are moving downwards. When there are slight irritation of signs in the bladder, that indicates the stones may be in the area of ureteral orifice in the bladder. If there is obvious irritation of signs in the bladder, weak stream of urine, interrupted and painful urination, it shows that the stones may have been moved to the bladder or posterior urethra. If a colicky pain remains continuously without any relief, it means that the treatment is not effective.

The Course of Treatment: A whole course of the general offensive therapy consists of 6 – 7 treatments, twice a week. If the stones descend but are not expelled or not totally expelled, then a second course can follow. The interval between two courses should be one to two weeks.

Points for Attention: After being treated by the general attack therapy, if the stones have not moved out and the patient is strong, some Chinese potent and dispersing drugs such as *Squama Manitis*, *Rhizoma Sparganii*, *Rhizoma Zedoariae*, *Radix Salviae Miltiorrhizae*, *Spina Gleditsiae*, *Resina Olibani*, *Myrrha* and others can be used. And then use general attack therapy, it is advisable to take measures of traditional Chinese medicine with western medicine to improve the patients' general conditions. If dihydrochlorothiazide and other diuretics have bee repeatedly taken, 1 gram of potassium chloride should be taken 3 times a day. After the general attack therapy, the patient may have symptoms like fatigue, loss of appetite, dizziness, then some drugs for supplementing qi, invigorating the spleen and nourishing the blood should be used to relieve them. After taking these drugs for 3 – 5 days, the patient will recover.

3. Simple Recipes and Proved Recipes

1) Recipe: *Modified Stone Expelling Decoction*

Endothelium Corneum Gigeriae Galli	15 g
Fructus Liquidambaris	15 g
Radix Linderae	15 g
Radix Salviae Miltiorrhizae	15 g
Semen Vaccariae	15 g
Rhizoma Alismatis	15 g

Concha Haliotidis	30 g
Folium Pyrrosiae	30 g
Talcum	30 g

Modification: For stasis of blood, *Spina Gleditsiae*, *Squama Manitis*, *Herba Lycopodii*, at 10 g each are added. For stagnancy of qi, *Fructus Aurantii*, *Fructus Foeniculi*, at 10 g each are added. For deficiency of qi, *Radix Astragali seu Hedysari*, *Radix Codonopsis Pilosulae*, at 15 g each are added; in severe case, *Radix Ginseng* 10 g is added. For deficiency of qi falling in the lower jiao, Buzhong yiqi tang is used with modifications. For deficiency of spleen, *Rhizoma Dioscoreae* 15 g, *Rhizoma Atractylodis Macrocephalae*, *Poria*, at 10 g each are added. For deficiency of blood, *Radix Angelicae Sinensis* 15 g, *Fructus Lycii*, *Radix Rehmanniae* at 10 g each are added. For deficiency of kidney yin, Erzhi wan, Liuwei dihuang wan or Shenqi wan are added. For deficiency of kidney yang, *Fructus Psoraleae*, *Radix Astragali Complanati*, *Radix Aconiti Praeparata*, at 10 g each are added. For colic or ache, *Radix Notoginseng*, *Succinum*, *Rhizoma Corydalis*, *Resina Olibani*, *Radix Saussureae Lappae*, *Radix Schefflerae Arboricolae*, at 10 g each and *Lignum Dalbergiae Odoriferae* 5 g are selected. For oliguria, *Rhizoma Imperatae*, *Semen Coicis*, at 15 each and *Medulla Tetrapanacis*, *Medulla Junci*, *Semen Malvae Vertillatae*, *Radix Stephaniae Tetrandrae*, *Polyporus Umbellatus*, at 10 g each are chosen. For hematuria, *Cacumen Biotae*, *Nodus Nelumbinis Rhizomatis*, *Herba Gephalanoploris*, *Herba Agrimoniae*, at 10 each are picked. For hydronephrosis, *Radix Astragali seu Hedysari*, *Radix Stephaniae Tetrandrae*, *Rhizoma Imperatae*, at 15 g individually are selected. For complication of infection, *Herba Violae*, *Herba Taraxaci*, at 15 g individually; *Fructus Gardeniae*, *Radix Pulsatillae*, *Herba Hedyotis Diffusae*, at 10 g each are picked.

Administration: Drugs are decocted with water. The decoction is taken at one dose a day in two portions in the morning and at night respectively. One course of treatment consisting of thirty days. A continuation of three courses is advised.

Among 1,001 cases treated with the above methods, 699 cases got recovery (of which 167 had their stones dissolved, 502 had their stones expelled.), 106 cases had their stones dissolved or partly expelled, 68 cases gained effectiveness. The total effective rate amounted to 84.3%.

2) *Ya Jiao Tong Instant Granules*

Formula of drugs: *Yajiaotong* is the extract of radix and cortex of *ginko tree*. Each packet is 10 g in weight, equivalent to crude drug 60 g.

Administration: Granules are swallowed with 150 – 200 ml of warm water at one packet b.i.d. Thirty days consisted of one course. For ureterolithiasis, three courses are necessary, for renal calculi, six courses are necessary.

In 176 cases treated clinically, 130 cases had their calculi expelled, 15 had their calculi moved downwards. The total effective rate is 82.39%. The biggest dimension of the calculus expelled is $2.0 \times 1.0 \times 1.0$ cm.

3) **Recipe:** *Regulating Middle and Eliminating Stone Decoction*

Radix Astragali seu Hedysari	30 g
Herba Lysimachiae	30 g
Rhizoma Cyperi	15 g
Fructus Citri	6 g
Spora Lygodii (to be wrapped)	15 g
Folium Pyrrosiae	12 g
Herba Polygoni Avicularis	12 g
Semen Plantaginis (to be wrapped)	15 g
Lignum Aquilariae Resinatum	10 g
Endothelium Corneum Gigeriae Galli	10 g
Natrii Sulphas	10 g
Mudella Tetrapanacis	6 g
Herba Chelidonii	3 g

Modification: For stagnancy of qi and stasis of blood, *Radix Rubiae*, *Herba Cephalanoploris*, *Radix Sanguisorbae*, *Herba Leonuri*, at 10 g each are added. For weak spleen and stomach, *Radix Dipsaci*, *Radix Codonopsis Pilosulae*, at 20 g each are added. For insufficiency of kidney, *Carapax Trionycis* 30 g, *Cortex Lycii Radicis*, *Rhizoma Aremarrhenae*, at 10 g each are added. For insufficiency of kidney yang, *Radix Dipsaci*, *Radix Aconiti Praeparata*, at 10 g each are added.

Administration: All the above drugs are to be decocted in water for oral administration. The decoction is given at one dose a day.

120 cases were treated clinically with a curative rate of 71.67% and a total effective rate of 98.33%.

4) **Recipe:** *Decoction for Treating Strangury and Expelling Stone*

Herba Lysimachiae	50 g
Spora Lygodii	25 g
Semen Plantaginis	20 g
Talcum	20 g
Folium Pyrrosiae	20 g
Rhizoma Alismatis	15 g
Herba Polygoni Avicularis	15 g
Caulis Clematidis Armandii	15 g
Radix Glycyrrhizae	10 g
Radix Aucklandiae	5 g

Modification: For qi stagnancy, *Fructus Aurantii Immaturus*, *Cortex Magnoliae Officinalis*, *Rhizoma Corydalis*, *Fructus Meliae Toosendan*, at 10 g each are added. For blood stasis, *Semen Persicae*, *Rhizoma Sparganii*, *Rhizoma Zedoariae*, *Squama Manitis*, *Faeces Trogopterori*, at 10 g each are added. For deficiency of kidney yin, *Radix Rehmanniae*, *Herba Cistanchis*, *Radix Ophiopogonis*, at 10 g each are added. For damp-heat, *Flos Lonicerae*, *Cortex Phellodendri*, *Fructus Forsythiae*, at 10 g each and *Herba Taraxaci* 15 g are added. For deficiency of kidney yin, *Radix Aconiti Praeparata*, *Radix Morindae Officinalis*, at 10 g each and *Cortex Cinnamomi* 5 g are added.

Administration: All the above drugs are to be decocted in water for oral administration. The decoction is taken at one dose a day. Synthetic drugs can also be used auxiliarily. Before taking medicine, the patients are advised to drink plenty of water. 20 mg of progesterone is injected intramuscularly b. i. d. for a continuation of ten days (a course of treatment). 20 ml of 25% magnesium sulfate is dissolved in 100 ml of 10% glucose saline for intravenous instillation which will be completed in twenty minutes. Later, 500 ml of 20% mannitose is instilled intravenously. It is to be completed in two hours. Treatment is given once a day. 7 to 10 days consisted of one course of treatment.

The above methods are used in treating 270 cases. Among the cases, 182 were cured, 71 were effective. The total effective rate accounted for 94.2%. The average hospitalization period was 12.5 days.

Acupuncture and Moxibustion

body acupuncture

Acupoints: **Shènshū**(BL23), **Pángguāngshū**(BL28), **Zúsānlǐ**(ST36) and **Guānyuán** (RN4).

Adjunct Points: **Zhōngjí**(RN3), **Sānyīnjiāo**(SP6), **Yīnlíngquán**(SP9), **Shuǐdào** (ST28).

Manipulation: Select 2 or 3 points each time and use strong stimulation. Do it twice a day, during which retain the needle for 20 – 30 minutes.

2) **Electrotherapy**

Acupoints: The cathode is connected with **Shènshū**(BL23) or **Pángguāngshū** (BL28), while the anode with **Guānyuán**(RN4) or **Shuǐdào**(ST28).

Manipulation: Select the upper and the lower points of the affected side for needling. The intensity of the needling should be from weak to strong and it must be as strong as the patient can bear. Then, sustain the needling for 20 – 30 minutes, once or twice a day.

Medicated Diet

1) Recipe: *Decoction of Lysimachia and Chicken's Gizzard*

Herba Lysimachiae	50 g
chicken's gizzard	2 set

Place the two ingredients in a small earthenware pot, pour cold water into the pot until the drugs are inundated; then stew them over soft fire for an hour.

To be taken twice a day, 300 ml of the soup and one chicken's gizzard each time. The soup is to be drunk and the gizzard taken along with bread or rice after being cut into slices and dipped in soy sauce, 15 to 30 days making up one course of treatment.

Recipe: *Decoction of Corn Stigma and Cogongrass Rhizome*

Stigma Maydis	30 g
Rhizoma Imperatae	30 g
Fructus Ziziphi Jujubae	8

Put all the three ingredients in a small aluminum pan with 1,500 ml of cold water and cook them over soft fire for 30 to 40 minutes.

To be taken twice a day, 500 ml each time. The decoction is to be drunk and the dates to be eaten, one month making up one course of treatment. This prescription can lead up to the best result when taken by patients suffering from incipient urethral calculi or vesical calculi marked by dark urine, red blood cells in urine proved by uroscopy accompanied with hypertension.

Recipe: *Decoction of Stalk Pith of Sunflower*

Medulla Hellianthi Annui	50 g
Talcum	10 g
Mel	1 spoonful

Decoct in 1,000 ml of cold water the first two ingredients in an earthenware pot; when the liquid is boiled down to 300 ml, sift the decoction from the dregs and mix honey into it.

To be taken as a drink every day. This recipe can treat strangury and is good for diuresis, and what is more, it has no side effect. It can also relieve summer-heat when drunk in summer.

Recipe: *Drink of Climbing Fern Spore and Tea*

Spora Lygodii	15 g
Folium Camelliae Viride	2 g

Infuse both of them n boiling water in a glass.

Take one glass first before meals after getting up every morning, then take it any time as you want to. Two months make up one course of treatment.

All the recipes stated above are applicable to the type of stagnation of damp-heat; those who suffer from stone of urinary system can choose any of them to eat.

Chapter Seven
Chronic Prostatitis

Chronic Prostatitis is a very common disease of the urinary system in the young and middle-aged male patients, far more common than the acute cases. With complicated clinical symptoms, it is hard to cure. The disease is usually a secondary infection of acute prostatitis or posterior urethritis. Sometimes, it may also be a secondary infection of the upper respiratory tract or mouth cavity. The familiar pathogens are *staphylococcus*, *streptococcus*, *colibacillus*, etc.. It is often induced by excessive alcoholic drinking, injury of the perineum, excessive sexual intercourses. According to usually-seen white secretion from the urethra, this disease falls into the categories of *Jīngzhuó* (turbid sperm) and *Láolìn* (*stranguria induce d by overstrain*) *in traditional Chinese medicine*.

ETIOLOGY AND PATHOGENESIS

The "door of essence room" is unlocked because of excessive sexual intercourse. Damp-heat takes the opportunity to occupy the room, forcing sperm to flow to the urinary bladder and leave the body along with urine. Then, there will result deficiency of the kidney-yin, hyperactivity of the ministerial fire, disturbance of essence room and retention of fire, all of which get together to lead to stagnation of *qi* and *blood* in the spermatic duct and cause this disease at last. If the disease course is prolonged, the deficient *yin* will involve *yang*. At this time, there will occur syndrome due to insufficiency of the kidney-*yang*.

MAIN SYMPTOMS AND SIGNS

White and turbid drip from the urethral meatus commonly seen at the end of urination or in the course of having a bowel movement with one's strength, or white sticky secretion from the urethral meatus usually found after getting up in the morning; frequent urination and burning urine and stabbing and itching urethra existing in most cases; tenesmus and distention and pain in the lower abdomen, lumbosacral portion, perineum and testes; listlessness, acraturesis, dizziness, insomnia, sexual hypoesthesia, spermatorrhea, prospermia, impotence and hemospermia.

MAIN POINTS OF DIAGNOSIS

1. Symptoms

1) **Urinary Symptoms:** There is frequent and urgent micturition, pain in micturition and an uncomfortable urination or a burning felling in micturition. At the end of urination or in moving the bowels, there is some sticky liquid dripping from the urethra.

2) **Pain:** There is a dull or a distending pain in the perineum and inside the rectum. The pain may radiate to the lumbosacral portion, the hip, the thigh, the testicle, the groin, etc..

3) **Disturbance of Sexual Function:** It is marked by sexual hypoesthesia, impotence, prospermia, pain in ejaculation, hemospermia, nocturnal emission, etc..

4) **Constitutional Symptoms:** There are neurasthenic symptoms such as weakness and fatigue in the whole body, aching pain at the waist and the back, insomnia, dreaminess, etc.. Sometimes, diseases such as arthritis, endocarditis, iritis, conjunctivitis and peripheral neuritis may be initiated.

2. Examination

1) **Rectal Examination:** This examination elicits a swollen prostate with tumefaction and obvious tenderness. Sometimes, the prostate may be hard and smaller than the usual size. The surface may be uneven and feels as if there are nodes on it. But it can also be normal at times.

2) **Examination of Prostatic Fluid:** Massage the prostate to collect prostatic fluid and examine it through microscopy. In a serious case there will be a lot of pus cells and more than 10 white cells being present in each high power field. On the other hand, the lecithin corpuscles will obviously decrease or disappear.

3) **The Three – glass Urine Test:** If there are pus cells in the first glass and

none in the second and the third glass or there pus cells in the first and the third glass and none in the second that means the infection probably comes from the prostate.

Bacterial Culture: After douching to sterilize and clean the urethra, massage prostate to collect the prostatic fluid for bacterial culture.

5) Use smear examination to find bacteria.

DIFFERENTIATION AND TREATMENT OF COMMON SYNDROMES

1. External Treatment

1) fumigation and washing therapy

(1) *Jiedu xiyao* is decocted in water for the decoction and hip bath is taken in this hot decoction to wash the perineum, 30 minutes each time, twice daily. This may be done with *Huoxue zhitong san* in the same way. The former is for the treatment of syndrome due to damp-heat, while the latter for syndrome due to stagnation of *qi* and *blood*.

Recipe: *Jiedu xiyao*

Herba Taraxaci	30 g
Radix Sophorae Flavescentis	12 g
Cortex Phellodendri	12 g
Fructus Forsythiae	12 g
Semen Momordicae	12 g
Flos Lonicerae	9 g
Radix Angelicae Dahuricae	9 g
Radix Paeoniae Rubra	9 g
Cortex Moutan Radicis	9 g
Radix Glycyrrhizae	9 g

The affected part of a patient's body is washed and fumed with the hot decoction, once or twice daily, 3 minutes each time.

Recipe: *Huoxue zhitong san*

Herba Speranskia Tuberculatae

Fructus Toosendan

Radix Angelicae Sinensis
Rhizoma Curcumae Longae
Fructus Corni
Rhizoma Dioscoreae
Cortex Moutan Radicis
Rhizoma Alismatis
Poria
Radix Aconiti Lateralis Praeparata
Semen Plantaginis
Rhizoma Achyranthis Bidentatae

(2) Put 15 grams of *Cortex Phellodendri*, 15 grams of *Alumen Exsiccatum* and 15 grams *Radix Salviae Miltiorrhizae* together and decoct them in water. Let the boiling decoction cool for 15 minutes till its temperature drops down to 42℃, then take a sitz bath for 10 – 15 minutes. Do this twice a day.

2) navel mounting therapy

First of all, take 0.15 grams of *Moschus* powder and put it into the navel. Then, grind 7 grains of *Fructus Piperis Albi* into fine powder and put it on top of the musk powder. Cover them with a piece of white paper (cut into a circular size just large enough to cover the navel), then fix the paper with a piece of adhesive plaster. Keep it for 7 – 10 days as a treatment and then change the dressing. A course consists of 10 times of treatment.

3) Have the infective substance discharged out of the prostate by massage of it so as to promote the absorption of the inflammation, once a week.

2. Internal Treatment

1) stasis – stagnancy type

Main Symptoms and Signs: The course of the sickness lasts for a long period with pain as the main affliction especially in the perineal region, sometimes involving the testis and the penis. In addition, it can even expand to the waist and the lower abdomen. The prostate gland will become hard and smaller than usual, accompanied by nodes. The prostatic fluid will not be easy to be collected or red blood cells can be found in it. The tongue is normal or with ecchymoses in it with thin and white fur. The pulse is thready and uneven.

Therapeutic Principles: Promote *blood* circulation, remove *blood* stasis and promote the flow of qi to remove stagnancy.

Recipe: *Qianliexianyan tang*

Radix Salviae Miltiorrhizae	9 g
Herba Lycopodii	9 g
Radix Paeoniae Rubra	9 g
Semen Persicae	9 g
Flos Carthami	9 g
Semen Vaccariae	9 g
Pericarpium Citri Reticulatae Viride	9 g
Radix Angelicae Dahuricae	9 g
Fructus Meliae Toosendan	9 g
Fructus Forsythiae	9 g
Herba Patriniae	15 g
Resina Olibani Praeparata	9 g
Myrrha Praeparata	9 g
Herba Taraxaci	30 g

All the above drugs are to be decocted in water for oral administration.

Modification: For hematuria and hemospermia, the drug added is *Radix Notoginseng* (in the form of powder and taken twice after being infused with water) 3 g. In case of harder prostata, the drugs added are *Squama Manitis Praeparata* 10 g, *Rhizoma Sparganii* 10 g and *Rhizoma Curculiginis* 10 g.

2) **damp - heat type**

Main Symptoms and Signs: The course of this sickness is comparatively short, usually accompanied with frequent, urgent and painful micturition, an uncomfortable or a burning feeling during urination. At the end of urination or in moving the bowels there is some whitish and turbid secretion dripping from the urethra. There is pain in the perineum, lumbosacral area, testis, etc.. In the prostatic fluid there are pus cells. The tongue is red with yellow greasy fur and the pulse is slippery and rapid.

Therapeutic Principles: Clear away pathogenic heat and dampness to treat secretion coming from the urethra.

Recipe: *San miao wan jiajian*

Cortex Phellodendri	15 g
Herba Patriniae	15 g
Rhizoma Atractylodis	10 g
Talcum	10 g
Rhizoma Alismatis	10 g
Rhizoma Dioscoreae Septemlobae	10 g
Herba Taraxaci	30 g
Rhizoma Achyranthis Bidentatae	20 g

All the above drugs are to be decocted in water for oral administration.

Recipe: *Bixie fenqing yin*

Rhizoma Dioscoreae Septemlobae	15 g
Semen Plantaginis	15 g
Herba Taraxaci	30 g
Herba Lycopodii	15 g
Herba Patriniae	30 g
Radix Paeoniae Rubra	15 g
Cortex Phellodendri	10 g
Poria	10 g
Rhizoma Alismatis	10 g
Radix Cyathulae	10 g
Fructus Gardeniae	10 g
Caulis Clematidis Armandii	6 g
Fructus Toosendan	10 g
Radix Glycyrrhizae	6 g

All the above drugs are to be decocted in water for oral administration.

3) kidney-deficiency type

Main Symptoms and Signs: After being ill for a long time, the patient will be very weak and fatigued and there will be an aching pain in the waist and in the legs, insomnia and dreaminess, listlessness, disturbance of sexual function, reddish tongue with little fur, thready and deep pulse.

Therapeutic Principles: Warming the kidney, supplementing qi, removing and dissolving pathogenic dampness and heat.

Recipe:

Rhizoma Curculiginis	15 g

Herba Epimedii	15 g
Rhizoma Dioscoreae	15 g
Herba Pyrrosiae	15 g
Cortex Phellodendri	9 g
Radix Angelicae Sinensis	9 g
Fructus Corni	9 g
Cortex Eucommiae	9 g
Herba Cistanchis	9 g
Radix Morindae Officinalis	9 g
Semen Allii Tuberosi	9 g
Actinolitum	30 g
Cortex Cinnamomi	3 g

All the above drugs are to be decocted in water for oral administration.

Modification: For those who have a great number of pus cells in the prostatic fluid, add 30 grams of *Herba Taraxaci*, 20 grams of *Semen Coicis* and 15 grams of *Herba Violae*. For those with severe pain in the waist, add 9 grams each of *Radix Dipsaci* and *Ramulus Loranthi*. For those with pain in the perineum, lower abdomen and the scrotum, increase the dosage of *Cortex Cinnamomi* up to 9 grams, and add 12 grams of *Fructus Meliae Toosendan*, 9 grams of *Rhizoma Cyperi* and *Fructus Forsythiae*. For those who are marked by frequency, urgency and pain in micturition, add 15 grams of *Talcum*, 30 grams of *Semen Phaseoli*, 9 grams each of *Herba Polygoni Avicularis* and *Herba Dianthi*.

4) syndrome due to hyperactivity of fire resulting from deficiency of *yin*

Main Symptoms and Signs: Soreness and weakness of the loins and knees, vertigo, insomnia, dreaminess, spermatorrhea, tendency of erecting of the penis, white turbid drip from the meatus urinarius at the end of urination or during the desire for sexual intercourse or in the course of having a bowel movement, or hemospermia, reddened tongue, and thready rapid pulse.

Therapeutic Principles: Nourish kidney-*yin* and purging ministerial *fire*

Recipe: Zhibai dihuang tang jiajian and Bixie fenqing yin

Radix Rehmanniae Praeparata	30 g
Rhizoma Alismatis	15 g
Rhizoma Dioscoreae Septemlobae	15 g
Semen Euryales	15 g

Rhizoma Anemarrhenae	10 g
Fructus Corni	12 g
Poria	10 g
Cortex Moutan Radicis	10 g
Cortex Phellodendri	10 g
Radix Saposhinkoviae	10 g
Semen Plantaginis	10 g
Rhizoma Achyranthis Bidentatae	

ction, which is taken warm in the morning and evening, one dose daily.

5) syndrome due to insufficiency of kidney – *yang*

Main Symptoms and Signs: Soreness and cold of the loins and knees, impotence, prospermia, spermatorrhea, frequent urination, dizziness, white turbid drips from the meatus urinarius due to mild strain, enlarged tender tongue with white coating, and deep thready pulse.

Therapeutic Principles: Reinforce the kidney, strengthen *yang*, control spermatorrhea and stop dribbling of the turbid from the meatus urinarius.

Recipe: *Jinsuo gujing wan* and *Yougui wan*

Semen Astragali Complanati	30 g
Radix Rehmanniae Praeparata	30 g
Semen Euryales	30 g
Os Draconis Fossilia	15 g
Concha Ostreae	15 g
Fructus Corni	15 g
Fructus Lycii	12 g
Rhizoma Achyranthis Bidentatae	12 g
Cortex Eucommiae Carbonisatus	12 g
Semen Cuscutae	12 g
Cortex Cinnamomi	10 g
Colla Cornus Cervi	10 g

All the above drugs are to be decocted in water for oral administration.

Massage

Press and knead **Shènshū(BL23), Mìngmén(DU4)** and **Yāoyángguān(DU3)** 30 times each, scrub **Yāoyǎn**(EX-B7) 30 times, thump the lumbar region 30 times, strike digitally **Guānyuán**(RN4) and **Zhōngjí**(RN3) 30 times each, rub Dantian clockwise and counterclockwise 30 times respectively, press-knead **Zúsānlǐ** (ST36), **Qūquán**(LR8) and **Sānyīnjiāo**(SP6) 30 times each and grasp **Yīnlíngquán** (SP9) and **Yánglíngquán**(GB34) 20 times each.

Modification: For patients with chronic prostatitis accompanied with soreness and distending pain of the loins, and pain, distention and tenesmus in the perineal, anal and suprapubic regions, press digitally **Huìyīn**(RN1) 30 times, grasp-pinch he medial muscle group 10 times and press-knead **Tàichōng**(LR3) and **Tàixī**(KI3) 30 times each.

For chronic prostatitis characterized by hesitant, frequent and dripping urination, whitish urine and itching discomfort in the urethra, press-knead **Píshū** (BL20) 30 times; scrub the lower abdomen 30 times, scrub horizontally the lumbosacral portion 30 times and press-knead **Tàixī**(KI3) and **Kūnlún**(BL60) 30 times each.

For chronic prostatitis with dizziness, insomnia, amnesia and asthenia, press-knead **Fēngchí**(GB20), **Bǎihuì**(DU20), **Píshū**(BL20), **Wèishū**(BL21), **Nèiguān** (PC6), **Shènshū**(BL23) and **Tàixī**(KI3) 30 times each.

For that accompanied with impotency, emission and premature ejaculation, press-knead **Zhìshì**(BL52) 30 times, scrub horizontally the lumbosacral portion 30 times and press-knead **Tàichōng**(LR3) and **Tàixī**(KI3) 30 times each.

Chapter Eight
Hyperplasia of Prostate

Hyperplasia of Prostate, also known as prostatic hyperplasia, is a very common disease that occurs in old male patients. Generally, this disease is considered to be associated with the disturbance of sexual hormones. The main manifestations are uroschesis and difficulty of urination. It belongs to the category of "Lóngbì" (retention of urine) in traditional Chinese medicine.

ETIOLOGY AND PATHOGENESIS

The urinary bladder works as if it were a state officer in charge of the storage of water. When it is in good condition, urination will be normal. Dysfunction of it leads to uroschesis. So the pathologic change of hyperplasia of prostate takes place in the urinary bladder. However, normal smooth urination is dependent on the normal function of *san jiao* and the normal function of *san jiao* relies on the lung, spleen and kidney. For instance, dysfunction of the lung (the upper − *jiao*) in descending makes water passages fail to be drained, which prevents water from flowing to the bladder. Disorder of the spleen and stomach (the middle − *jiao*) leads to accumulation of damp − heat in the bladder or weakness of the spleen − *qi* brings about sinking of the *qi* of the middle − *jiao* to the bladder, either of which troubles the bladder. In addition, deficiency of the *qi* of the kidney (the lower − *jiao* results in imbalance between *yin* and *yang*, which also influences the bladder. In short, disturbance of any of above organs will, in the end, cause anuresis, uneven urination, enuresis and urinary incontinence. Moreover, symptoms such as anuresis may be induced due to accumulation of *blood* in the bladder, for the *blood* stasis will block water passages.

MAIN SYMPTOMS AND SIGNS

Slow onset, frequent urination occurring at the early stage which is especially obvious at night, difficulty in urination appearing after the symptom frequent urination, urination taking place after long waiting, dribbling of urine at the end of the urination which gives the feeling that the urination is not complete. Urinating in fraction because of incomplete urination, urination becoming more difficult as the obstruction is getting ever so severe, urinating within short range, thin urine scream, more and more urine retained in the bladder which is often distended so as to cause chronic uroschesis, even voluntary micturition (false urinary incontinence) or enuresis at night, great amount of hematuria occasionally seen when the superficial cirsoid phleborrhexis of the glands occurs, stone and hyperemia of the prostata and the neck of the bladder and symptoms due to acute uroschesis or irritation to the bladder all of which are induced by overstrain, affection of cold, excess of sexual intercourse, over – intake of pungent or irritant food or secondary infection of the bladder, high blood pressure, acratia, dizziness, vertigo, poor appetite, and complications of pile, hernia, proctoptosis and hematochezia.

MAIN POINTS OF DIAGNOSIS

1. It occurs mostly in aged people over 50.
2. 2. **Symptoms**

1) *Frequent Micturition*: This is a symptom at the early stage of the disease. Gradually, the frequency of urination increases, which is obvious especially at night. In mild cases the urination will happen 4 – 5 times a night and in severe cases it may occur dozens of times.

2) *Difficulty in Urination*: At the beginning, the patient has to wait for a while before urination. Later on, the obstructive condition becomes more severe, accompanied with difficulty in urination, weak and thready stream of urine, then interruption or even dribbling in urination.

3) *Acute Uroschesis*: This symptom is due to factors such as constipation, cold, alcoholic drinking and weariness which can cause hyperemia and hydrops of the neck of the urinary bladder. Complete obstruction may be formed and acute

uroschesis will result.

4) *Urinary Incontinencies* : When the filling of the urinary bladder reaches an extreme state and the intravesical pressure becomes higher than the resistance of the sphincter muscle of urethra, urine will dribble out continuously from the urethra. This phenomenon is called pseudo-uroschesis.

5) *Hematuria* : Because of the hyperemia of the neck of urinary bladder, sometimes, hematuria may be found under microscopy or even by gross inspection.

6) *Complications* : Urinary obstruction for a long time may lead to other sicknesses such as decrease of renal functions or even renal failure, manifested by loss of appetite, fatigue, then nausea and vomiting, hypertension and anemia. Finally, a coma will result. On the other hand, a long term difficulty in urination may also cause the increase of abdominal pressure and produce inguinal hernia, hemorrhoid, proctoptosis, varicose vein in the lower limbs and so on.

3. Examination

1) *Digital Examination of Rectum* : Prior to the examination, the contents in the urinary bladder should be entirely cleared out. The examination often shows that the prostate gland is larger than usual but its surface is smooth with no nodes on it. Its edge is distinct and the hardness is medium with resilience. The central sulcus becomes shallow or disappears.

2) *Residual Urinary Test* : The residual urine is the amount of remaining urine which is collected by urethral catheterization immediately after urination.

3) *Cystoscopy and Cystography* : If the middle lobe of the prostate increases in size, it is necessary to go through cystoscopy and cystography in order to confirm the diagnosis.

4) *Ultrasonic Examination* : This examination will show the volume, form and internal structure of the prostate gland.

5) *Laboratory Examination* : Through routine uroscopy, pus cells or red blood cells may be found. Prolonged urinary retention may influence the function of the kidney. Therefore, a further test of urea nitrogen and creatinine will be required.

DIFFERENTIATION AND TREATMENT OF COMMON SYNDROMES

1. External Treatment

1) external application

250 g of *Natrii Chloride* is parched warm and then wrapped in a piece of cloth, which is used to compress the lower abdomen, 30 minutes each time, twice daily. Remember to keep the *Natrii Chloride* warm through another parching.

2) massage

Have the patient lie on his back and extend his legs straight in the way of abduction and extorsion. Push the point **Jīmén(SP11)** of the right leg unidirectionally from the lower to the upper with an even forceful manipulation of moderate speed, 1,000 times are required in each treatment. In case of distending pain in the bladder due to long-time uroschesis, the two points of both legs are pushed simultaneously.

3) acupuncture therapy

The points **Zhōngjí (RN3)**, **Sānyīnjiāo (SP6)**, **Yīnlíngquán (SP9)** and **Pángguāngshū(BL28)** are punctured. In case of general weakness, moxibustion may be done over the points **Guānyuán(RN4)** and **Qìhǎi(RN6)**.

4) urethral catheterization

If there is no curative effects obtained from the above, urinary catheter is inserted to drain the urine with aseptic manipulation.

5) operative treatment

Operation should be considered for those refusing all the other therapies.

2. Internal Treatment

Anuresis, dribbling of urine and difficulty in urination are symptoms of excess type; urinary incontinence or enuresis, deficiency type; sudden anuresis, excess type; and long-time of anuresis, deficiency type. Symptoms of excess type are treated mainly through promoting diuresis, while deficiency type, through tonifying.

1) syndrome due to obstruction of water passage resulting from dysfunction of the lung

Main Symptoms and Signs: Uneven urination, even anuresis, dry throat and mouth, cough with sputum and dyspnea, thin yellow or white tongue coating and rapid pulse.

Therapeutic Principles: Promoting the flow of lung- qi, clearing away heat and inducing diuresis.

Recipe: *Huangqin qingfei yin*

Radix Scutellariae	12 g
Cortex Mori	12 g
Radix Ophiopogonis	12 g
Fructus Gardeniae	10 g
Caulis Clematidis Armandii	10 g
Radix Platycodi	10 g
Semen Armeniacae Amarum	10 g
Semen Plantaginis	15 g
Poria	12 g
Rhizoma Imperatae	30 g

All the above drugs are to be decocted in water for oral administration.

2) syndrome due to damp-heat descending to the urinary bladder

Main Symptoms and Signs: Uneven urination, yellowish and hot urine, itching and pain in the penis, even anuresis, spasm and distention of the lower abdomen, reddened tongue with yellow greasy coating, and slippery rapid pulse.

Therapeutic Principles: Clear away damp-heat from the urinary bladder.

Recipe: *Bazheng san*

Herba Polygoni Avicularis	15 g
Herba Dianthi	15 g
Semen Plantaginis	15 g
Spora Lygodii	15 g
Herba Taraxaci	30 g
Herba Lysimachiae	30 g

Cortex Phellodendri	10 g
Caulis Clematidis Armandii	10 g
Fructus Gardeniae	10 g
Radix et Rhizoma Rhei	10 g
Rhizoma Achyranthis Bidentatae	10 g
Radix Glycyrrhizae	10 g

All the above drugs are to be decocted in water for oral administration.

3) **syndrome due to irresponsible bladder resulting from sinking of the** qi of the middle-jiao

Main Symptoms and Signs: Urinary incontinence or enuresis, listlessness, shortness of breath, languor, pale complexion, pale tongue with white coating, and thready feeble pulse.

Therapeutic Principles: Reinforce the middle-jiao, invigorate qi and restrain the bladder.

Recipe: *Buzhong yiqi tang*

Radix Astragali seu Hedysari	30 g
Radix Codonopsis	15 g
Rhizoma Atractylodis Macrocephalae	12 g
Radix Angelicae Sinensis	12 g
Pericarpium Citri Reticulatae	10 g
Radix Bupleuri	10 g
Rhizoma Cimicifugae	10 g
Radix Glycyrrhizae	6 g
Fructus Rosae Laevigatae	15 g
Fructus Alpiniae Oxyphyllae	15 g

All the above drugs are to be decocted in water for oral administration.

4) **syndrome due to incomplete urination resulting from insufficiency of the kidney-** yin

Main Symptoms and Signs: Frequent urination with dribbling and retained urine, dizziness, vertigo, soreness and weakness of the loins and knees, dreaminess, insomnia; and reddened tongue, dry throat, yellowish hot urine and thready rapid pulse in cases with heat due to yin-deficiency.

Therapeutic Principles: Nourish the kidney-yin and activate the bladder.

Recipe: *Zhibai dihuang tang jiajian*

Rhizoma Anemarrhenae	12 g
Cortex Phellodendri	10 g
Radix Rehmanniae Praeparata	10 g
Rhizoma Alismatis	12 g
Poria	10 g
Cortex Moutan Radicis	10 g
Rhizoma Dioscoreae	12 g
Fructus Corni	10 g
Herba Dianthi	15 g
Herba Polygoni Avicularis	15 g
Rhizoma Achyranthis Bidentatae	10 g
Semen Plantaginis	

(decocted after being wrapped in a piece of cloth)

All the above drugs are to be decocted in water for oral administration.

5) **syndrome due to dysfunction of** *qi* resulting from insufficiency of the kidney-*yang*

Main Symptoms and Signs: Anuresis or dribbling urine, pale complexion, soreness and cold of the loins and knees, pale tongue with white coating, and deep thready slow feeble pulse.

Therapeutic Principles: Warm and reinforce the kidney-*yang* and remove obstruction to promote diuresis.

Recipe: *Jisheng shenqi wan*

Radix Rehmanniae Praeparata	20 g
Rhizoma Dioscoreae	15 g
Poria	15 g
Semen Plantaginis	15 g

(decocted after being wrapped in a piece of cloth)

Rhizoma Alismatis	12 g
Radix Aconiti Lateralis Praeparata	10 g
Cortex Cinnamomi	10 g
Rhizoma Achyranthis Bidentatae	10 g
Herba Cistanchis	10 g

All the above drugs are to be decocted in water for oral administration.

Hyperplasia of Prostate

6) **syndrome due to obstruction of the bladder resulting retention of blood in the lower** – *jiao*

Main Symptoms and Signs: Urinating with great efforts or anuresis, distending pain in the perineum and lower abdomen, occasional hematuria or hemospermia, dark purple or ecchymoses – dotted tongue, and thready taut uneven pulse.

Therapeutic Principles: Promote blood circulation, resolve mass and remove obstruction in the bladder.

Recipe:

Thallus Laminariae seu Echloniae	20 g
Sargassum	20 g
Spica Prunellae	15 g
Radix Rehmanniae Praeparata	15 g
Herba Verbenae	15 g
Herba Polygoni Avicularis	15 g
Herba Dianthi	15 g
Herba Lycopodii	15 g
Rhizoma Sparganii	10 g
Rhizoma Curcumae	10 g
Squama Manitis Praeparata	10 g
Semen Vaccariae	10 g
Rhizoma Achyranthis Bidentatae	10 g
Radix Glycyrrhizae	6 g

All the above drugs are to be decocted in water for oral administration.

Medicated Diet

Recipe: *Kidneys stewed with Eucommia bark*

sheep kidney	2
Cortex Eucommiae	15 g
Rhizoma Zingiberis Recens	right amount
Bulbus Allii Fistulosi	right amount
table salt	right amount

Cut the kidneys open, get rid of the membrane; then stew them together with all the other ingredients until the kidneys are done.

The kidneys are to be eaten. Applicable to patients suffering from prostatic hyperplasia of deficiency cold of the lower-jiao.

Recipe: *Decoction of Aniseed and Chinese Green Onion*

Fructus Forsythiae	5 g
Bulbus Allii Fistulosi	4

Pound them together and decoct them for oral administration. To be taken in three separate doses. Applicable to patients suffering from prostatic hyperplasia of deficiency-cold of lower- *jiao*.

Recipe: *Mung Bean Gruel*

Semen Phaseoli Radiati	80 g
Fructus Tritici	50 g
Medulla Tetrapanacis	10 g

Decoct the last ingredient in water and remove the dregs, and then make gruel with the decoction and the first two ingredients.

To be taken as breakfast. Applicable to patients suffering from prostatic hyperplasia of stagnation of damp-heat.

Chapter Nine
Epididymitis

Epididymitis is mainly due to infection of bacteria through the spermatic duct, usually originating from infection of urethra, prostata or seminal vesicle. Traditional Chinese medicine includes it in the category of Zǐyōng (acute or chronic orchitis and epididymitis).

ETIOLOGY AND PATHOGENESIS

Stagnation of *qi* and *blood* in the testis due to going down of damp-heat in the *Liver Meridian* and retention of noxious-damp-heat in the channels lead to this disease. Excessive heat due to long stagnation of *qi* and *blood* may turn flesh into pus. *Qi* and *blood* retained so long will Turn into chronic mass.

MAIN SYMPTOMS AND SIGNS

Sudden onset in acute cases, swelling and pain of the epididymis, the testis enlarged when it has been involved in the inflammation, red-swelling and burning-pain of the scrotum, dragging pain in the lower abdomen occurring when the inflammation involves the funiculus, red swollen bright skin of the scrotum whose center is soft and raised due to suppuration, the symptoms vanishing more rapidly and the sore healing gradually after incision or ulceration of the abscess which is followed by discharging of pus and purging of toxins, chills, fever, thirst, deep-colored urine, enlarged remarkedly tender epididymis and testis seen through examination, complications of funiculitis and hydrocele testis, and slightly tender or tenesmic distending cold-painful tough mass or hard node in the epididymis or testis of chronic cases.

MAIN POINTS OF DIAGNOSIS

Chronic epididymitis is to be differentiated from the following diseases.

1. tuberculosis of epididymis
Some symptoms at the early stage of this disease are similar to those of acute epididymitis. During the late stage, the tail of epididymis or the whole epididymis has become a hard node without severe tenderness. Cementing with the skin of scrotum, this hard node may involve the testis and have sinus. There are nodes like a string of beads in the spermatic duct. Hard nodes in the prostata and seminal vesicle may be palpable when digital examination of rectum is conducted.

2. cystis of epididymis
Tenser semi-transparent mass may occur in any part of the epididymis and located at the back of the testis.

3. Orchioncus
Enlarged, not painful, solid and heavier testis with node-like surface but without the original elasticity, possible distant transfer lymph nodes, and complications of hydrocele of tunica vaginalis and hematoma of scrotum.

DIFFERENTIATION AND TREATMENT OF COMMON SYNDROMES

1. External Treatment

1) the acute stage
Jinhuang gao or *Daqing gao* is externally applied to the local part. Incision for drainage should be conducted after suppuration. Routine dressing change is carried out according to that in treatment of pyogenic diseases after ulceration. Bed rest is suggested with the scrotum supported with bandage of scrotal support.

2) the chronic stage
30 g of *Chonghe gao fen* is infused with 300 ml of boiling water. The affected

part is soaked in, and washed with the medicated water, which is kept warm, 20 minutes each time, twice daily.

Recipe: *Chonghe gao*

Cortex Cercis Chinensis	150 g
Radix Angelicae Pubescentis	90 g
Radix Paeoniae Rubra	30 g
Radix Angelicae Dahuricae	30 g
Radix Acori Tatarinowii	45 g

2. Internal Treatment

1) the acute stage (syndrome due to damp – heat having gone down)

Main Symptoms and Signs: Red swollen burning painful tender epididymis and scrotum, chills, fever, thirst, yellowish urine, dry stools, yellow greasy tongue coating, and taut slippery rapid pulse.

Therapeutic Principles: Clear away heat from the liver, promote diuresis, remove toxic material and subduing swelling.

Recipe: *Longdan xiegan tang jiajian*

Radix Gentianae	10 g
Radix Bupleuri	10 g
Radix Scutellariae	10 g
Cortex Phellodendri	10 g
Fructus Gardeniae	10 g
Rhizoma Alismatis	10 g
Semen Citri Reticulatae	10 g
Radix Cyathulae	10 g
Radix Paeoniae Rubra	15 g
Herba Violae	20 g
Radix Isatidis	30 g
Flos Lonicerae	30 g
Caulis Clematidis Armandii	6 g

All the above drugs are to be decocted in water for oral administration.

Modification: In case of persistent high fever, the dosage of *Radix Bupleuri* and *Radix Scutellariae* in the original prescription is separately changed into 15 g, and 15 g of *Fructus Forsythiae* is added.

In case of constipation, 10 g of *Radix et Rhizoma Rhei* is added.

In case of severe swelling and pain, 1.5 – 3 g of *Xihuang wan* is infused in water and then taken. After suppuration, the drugs added are *Squama Manitis Praeparata* 10 g, *Spina Gleditsiae* 10 g.

2) the chronic stage (syndrome due to stagnation of *qi* and *blood*

Main Symptoms and Signs: Tough mass or hard node with mild tenderness in the affected part; tenesmus, distention, cold – pain in the lower abdomen; the swelling and pain probably aggravated by overstrain or pungent food, white tongue coating, and thready taut pulse.

Therapeutic Principles: Soothe the liver, regulate *qi*, remove *blood* stasis and disperse mass.

Recipe: *Gouju tang*

Fructus Citri Reticulatae	10 g
Fructus Toosendan	10 g
Bombyx Batryticatus	10 g
Squama Manitis Praeparata	10 g
Semen Citri Reticulatae	10 g
Semen Litchi	10 g
Semen Crataegi	15 g
Rhizoma Achyranthis Bidentatae	10 g
Radix Linderae	10 g
Radix Bupleuri	10 g
Spica Prunellae	15 g
Thallus Laminariae seu Echloniae	15 g
Radix Paeoniae Rubra	20 g
Fructus Foeniculi	6 g
Radix Aconiti Lateralis Praeparata	6 g

All the above drugs are to be decocted in water for oral administration.

Modification: Together with the decoction, *Sanjie pian* is taken for the purpose of subduing swelling and resolving mass.

Chapter Ten
Tuberculosis of Epididymis

Tuberculosis of epididymis is one of the common tuberculoses of the reproductive system and a secondary disease of tuberculosis in other parts of the body. It is usually caused by infection due to invasion of *Myobacteria tuberculosis* into the epididymis through posterior urethra and spermatic duct. Modern traditional Chinese medicine physicians called this disease as Zĭtán according to the nature of líután (tuberculosis of bones and joints).

ETIOLOGY AND PATHOGENESIS

Phlegm takes the advantage of weakness of the vessels due to impairment of the liver and kidney to go downwards into the testis, where it stays and cause this disease. Heat is produced because of long retention of phlegm and pus comes from spoiled flesh due to excessive heat. In the course of suppuration, syndrome due to internal heat resulting from yin - deficiency may be caused by heat from phlegm. Manifestations due to $yang$ - deficiency of the kidney may also appear when long time of yin - deficiency has involved $yang$.

MAIN SYMPTOMS AND SIGNS

symptoms and signs

Common in the young and middle - aged of 20 - 35, slow development, a hard node usually occurring at the tail of unilateral epididymis and then diffusing to the whole epididymis and testis, the node with usual tenderness, mild pain or tenesmic distending pain, thickened funiculus, nodes like a string of beads existing in the spermatic duct, such presentations coming into being after months or years as cementation of masses in the testis with the skin, swelling gradually becoming obvious, dark - red skin and formation of abscess of cold nature, thin pus with necrotic tissue like bean dregs - like or caseous thing discharged after ulceration, unhealing sinus, no general symptoms usually at the early stage, and symptoms of internal heat due to *yin* - deficiency or *yang* - deficiency of the kidney probably appearing after suppuration and ulceration.

Examination

Slightly enlarged prostata and hard node seen in digital examination of rectum, higher lymphocyte count and accelerated blood sedimentation seen in blood test, red blood cells seen in microscopy of urine, and positive tuberculin test in most cases.

DIFFERENTIATION AND TREATMENT OF COMMON SYNDROMES

1. External Treatment

Yanghe jiening gao is applied at the early stage. Incision for drainage should be performed when pus fails to be absorbed. Dressing change is conducted, after ulceration, with drugs having the action of expelling pus and removing necrosis, but corrosive drugs should be cautiously used. Dressing change with drugs having the action of promoting the generation of tissue is suggested when necrosis is about to fall off and fresh tissue is going to generate.

2) During the early stage, ionotherapy may be tried locally. The diseased scrotum may be held with a scrotal support. If the sinus fails to respond to any treatment, operation should be considered.

2. Internal Treatment

the early stage

Main Symptoms and Signs: Not painful or slightly tenesmic - distending mass with normal skin and temperature, no remarkable general symptoms in most cases, white tongue coating, and deep thready pulse.

Therapeutic Principles: Tonify the liver and kidney, warm the channels, dredging the collateral, resolve phlegm and disperse mass.

Recipe: *Yanghe tang*

Radix Rehmanniae Praeparata	30 g
Herba Ephedrae	3 g
Colla Cornus Cervi	10 g
Semen Sinapis Album	10 g
Rhizoma Zingiberis Carbonisatus	6 g
Cortex Cinnamomi	6 g
Radix Glycyrrhizae	6 g
Rhizoma Achyranthis Bidentatae	12 g
Semen Citri Reticulatae	10 g
Radix Stemonae	10 g
Concha Ostreae	20 g
Radix Salviae Miltiorrhizae	15 g

All the above drugs are to be decocted in water for oral administration.

Modification: *Xiaojin dan* or *Sichong pian* may be taken together with the decoction.

2) the suppurative stage

Main Symptoms and Signs: Enlarged scrotum, cementation of mass in the testis with the skin which is dark red, slight fever, hectic fever, night sweat, feverish sensation in the palms and soles, reddened tongue with little coating, and thready rapid pulse.

Therapeutic Principles: Nourish yin, clear away heat, eliminate dampness, resolve phlegm and expel pus from within by eruption.

Recipe: *Ziyin chushi tang*

Radix Rehmanniae Praeparata	30 g
Radix Bupleuri	10 g
Radix Scutellariae	10 g
Cortex Lycii	10 g
Rhizoma Anemarrhenae	12 g
Bulbus Fritillariae Thunbergii	10 g
Rhizoma Alismatis	10 g
Radix Angelicae Sinensis	12 g
Rhizoma Achyranthis Bidentatae	12 g
Radix Astragali seu Hedysari	20 g

Squama Manitis Praeparata	10 g
Spina Gleditsiae	10 g

All the above drugs are to be decocted in water for oral administration.

3) **the postulcerative stage**

(1) *syndrome due to deficiency of* yang

Main Symptoms and Signs: Pus as thin as sputum, grey and dark granulation on the surface of the sore, pale complexion, cold limbs, chills, loose stools, frequent urination, enlarged tender tongue with white coating, and deep thready slow pulse.

Therapeutic Principles: Invigorate qi, nourish blood, drastically tonify the liver and kidney.

Recipe: Xiantian dazao tang jiajian

Radix Rehmanniae Praeparata	30 g
Radix Polygoni Multiflori	12 g
Herba Cistanchis	10 g
Rhizoma Curculiginis	10 g
Placenta Hominis	3 g
Semen Cuscutae	12 g
Rhizoma Polygonati	15 g
Fructus Lycii	10 g
Rhizoma Atractylodis Macrocephalae	12 g
Rhizoma Achyranthis Bidentatae	10 g
Radix Angelicae Sinensis	15 g
Radix Codonopsis	15 g
Poria	
Cortex Cinnamomi	3 g
Radix Astragali seu Hedysari	30 g
Radix Glycyrrhizae	6 g

All the above drugs are to be decocted in water for oral administration.

(2) *syndrome due to internal heat resulting from deficiency of* yin

Treatment is based on Ziyin chushi tang jiajian used during the suppurative stage.

Recipe: Ziyin chushi tang

Rhizoma Ligustici Chuanxiong
Radix Angelicae Sinensis
Radix Paeoniae Alba
Radix Rehmanniae Praeparata
Radix Bupleuri
Radix Scutellariae
Pericarpium Citri Reticulatae
Bulbus Fritillariae Thunbergii
Cortex Lycii
Rhizoma Alismatis
Radix Glycyrrhizae
Rhizoma Zingiberis Recens

Chapter Eleven
Hydrocele of Tunica Vaginalis

U_{nder} normal condition, balance between secretion and absorption of fluid in the capusle of tunica vaginalis testis is kept. When hypersecretion or hypoabsorption has been caused by some pathogenic factor, hydrocele of tunica vaginalis results. This disease falls into two types: congenital and secondary. The former is common in infants and very young children, while the latter in adults. As a common disease of scrotum, it is included in the category of Shuǐshàn (hydrocele) in traditional Chinese medicine.

ETIOLOGY AND PATHOGENESIS

That in infants and very young children is usually caused by retention of fluid in the scrotum due to inadequate functional activity of the kidney − qi resulting from congenital weakness. That in adults is often caused similar to this. Cold − dampness in the *Kidney Meridian* caused by affection of exogenous cold − dampness and retention of water due to sweating after overstrain, catching in the rain or long sitting on wet ground, damp − heat in the *Liver Meridian* and obstruction of blood stasis in the channels due to trauma or retention of water lead to water or damp − heat to go downwards to the scrotum and stay there to result in this disease.

MAIN SYMPTOMS AND SIGNS

Gradually enlarged unilateral scrotum with egg − shaped, smooth, cystic and not painful mass; tenesmus due to bigger mass, penis buried by the skin around due to too big mass which makes urination and sexual intercourse difficult, testis and epididymis impalpable because they are surrounded by hydrops, testis may be palpable in funicular hydrocele of tunica vaginalis because the mass is above the testis, congenital hydrocele of tunica vaginalis gradually reduced up to vanishing when the patient is in dorsal position, ordinary hydrocele of tunica vaginalis remaining the same even if the patient is in different position, and positive transillumination of the cystic mass in hydrocele of tunica vaginalis.

MAIN POINTS OF DIAGNOSIS

1. inguinal hernia

The mass capable of going into the abdominal cavity, bound of the mass sensed during coughing, no fluctuation, palpable testis, and negative transillumination.

2. congenital hydrocele of tunica vaginalis

The characteristics except positive transillumination are the same as those of hernia.

DIFFERENTIATION AND TREATMENT OF COMMON SYNDROMES

1. External Treatment

Recipe: *Proved recipe* 1

Galla Chinensis	30 g
Alumen	15 g
Fructus Foeniculi	10 g

The drugs are decocted in water for the decoction. The affected part is fumigated and then washed with the hot decoction twice daily.

Indications: Hydrocele of tunica vaginalis in infants and very young children.

Recipe: *Xiaofan xiyao*

Natrii Sulphas 12 g	
Borax	10 g
Alumen	10 g

The drugs are infused with boiling water, which is kept warm with heat. The affected part is fumigated and washed with warm water. One dose is used twice daily.

Indications: Hydrocele of tunica vaginalis with the syndrome due to damp-heat in the *Liver Meridian*.

Recipe: *Proved recipe* 2

Fructus Foeniculi	30 g
Semen Citri Reticulatae	30 g

The drugs are ground into rough powder, parched warm and put into a cloth bag. The scrotum is compressed with the hot bag, once daily.

Indications: Hydrocele of tunica vaginalis with the syndrome due to cold-dampness resulting from deficiency of the kidney.

Recipe: *Huoxue zhitong san*

Herba Aperanskiae Tuberculatae	30 g
Fructus Toosendan	15 g
Radix Angelicae Sinensis	15 g
Rhizoma Curcumae Longae	15 g
Cortex Erythrinae	15 g
Radix Clematidis	15 g
Radix Cyathulae	15 g
Rhizoma seu Radix Notopterygii	15 g
Radix Angelicae Dahuricae	15 g
Lignum Sappan	15 g
Cortex Acanthopanacis	15 g
Flos Carthami	15 g
Rhizoma Smilacis Glabrae	15 g
Pericarpium Zanthoxyli	6 g
Olibanum	6 g

The drugs are decocted in water. The affected part is fumigated and washed with the hot decoction, twice daily.

Indications: Hydrocele of tunica vaginalis with the syndrome due to accumulation of blood stasis.

Recipe: *Proven prescription*

Fructus Foeniculi	1 - 3 g

duck's egg with green shell	one
Sodium Chloride	small amount
Oleum Arachidis	proper amount

Fructus Foeniculi is parched up to brown and then ground into very fine powder, which is mixed in an iron pot with *Sodium Chloride*, *Oleum Arachidis* and the *duck's eggs* with the shells removed, into a mixture. The mixture is stir-fried until it is well done and then taken at a draught. This is done once daily.

6) **operative treatment**

Very big mass in the scrotum or mass having been treated with drugs for over one month but without curative effects should be given an operation.

2. Internal Treatment

1) **treatment for infants and very young children**

Main Symptoms and Signs: Chills, cold limbs, pale complexion, shortness of breath, languor, frequent urination, pale tongue with white coating, and deep thready pulse.

Therapeutic Principles: Warm the kidney, activate *yang*, promote the flow of *qi* and induce diuresis.

Jisheng shenqi wan is applied. 1–3 g of the pills taken with water each time, twice or three times daily.

2) **treatment for adults**

(1) *syndrome due to cold-dampness resulting from deficiency of the kidney*

Main Symptoms and Signs: Dampness and cold of the scrotum, cold-pain of the loins and knees, clear and profuse urine, pale tongue with white greasy coating, and deep thready pulse.

Therapeutic Principles: Warming the kidney, dispelling cold, promoting diuresis and subduing swelling.

Recipe: *Baojian danggui sini tang* and *Daoqi tang*

Radix Angelicae Sinensis	12 g
Radix Aconiti Lateralis Praeparata	10 g
Fructus Foeniculi	6 g

Cortex Cinnamomi	10 g
Radix Linderae	10 g
Radix Bupleuri	10 g
Radix Paeoniae Rubra	10 g
Rhizoma Corydalis	10 g
Fructus Toosendan	10 g
Semen Plantaginis	10 g
Poria	15 g
Rhizoma Alismatis	15 g

All the above drugs are to be decocted in water for oral administration. Taken warm in the morning and evening, one dose daily.

(2) **syndrome due to damp – heat in** Liver Meridian

Main Symptoms and Signs: Damp and hot scrotum, swollen and painful testis and epididymis, yellowish urine, yellow and greasy tongue coating, and taut slippery rapid pulse.

Therapeutic Principles: Clear away heat from the liver, promoting diuresis and subduing swelling.

Recipe: Longdan xiegan tang

Radix Gentianae	10 g
Radix Scutellariae	10 g
Fructus Gardeniae	10 g
Rhizoma Alismatis	12 g
Radix Rehmanniae	15 g
Radix Bupleuri	10 g
Semen Plantaginis	10 g

(decocted after being wrapped in a piece of cloth)

Radix Angelicae Sinensis	10 g
Radix Glycyrrhizae	3 g
Caulis Clematidis Armandii	6 g

All the above drugs are to be decocted in water for oral administration.

(3) **syndrome due to accumulation of blood stasis**

Main Symptoms and Signs: Swollen and painful scrotum with dark purple skin, negative transillumination in most cases, purplish tongue with white coating, and taut uneven pulse.

Therapeutic Principles: Promote blood circulation to remove blood stasis, induce diuresis to subdue swelling.

Recipe: *Huoxue sanyu tang jiajian*

Radix Angelicae Sinensis	15 g
Radix Paeoniae Rubra	15 g
Semen Persicae	10 g
Rhizoma Ligustici Chuanxiong	10 g
Radix et Rhizoma Rhei	6 g
Cortex Moutan Radicis	10 g
Rhizoma Achyranthis Bidentatae	12 g
Herba Lycopodii	15 g
Rhizoma Alismatis	15 g
Polyporus	15 g
Radix Glycyrrhizae	6 g

All the above drugs are to be decocted in water for oral administration.

Chapter Twelve
Induration of Penis

Induration of Penis refers to fibrosis of cavernous body of penis. It is due to fibrous masses produced between tunica albuginea corporum cavernosorsum and fascia penis.

ETIOLOGY AND PATHOGENESIS

qi and *blood* stagnated in the *Liver Meridian* and phlegm produced in the interior due to dysfunction of the spleen go downwards to the penis, where they accumulated and cause this disease. Because *Shaoyin* of the foot is connected with the penis, syndrome due to *yin* – deficiency of the liver and kidney may be seen sometimes.

MAIN SYMPTOMS AND SIGNS

This disease is common in middle – aged males and manifested by distinctly – bordered, usually fixed, hard cord – like or plaque – type nodes palpable on the dorsum penis. The nodes, in general, do not attract any attention but make the penis painful and bent when it has erected, influencing sexual life in severe cases. However, they do not disturb urination nor fester. Shadow of calcification or ossification may be seen in roentgenogram.

DIFFERENTIATION AND TREATMENT OF COMMON SYNDROMES

1. External Treatment

Local application of small pieces of *Yanghe jiening gao* is conducted with the dressing change taking place once a week. Or, audio frequency physiotherapy is carried out, once to twice each week, 10 times consisting of one course of treatment.

2. Internal Treatment

1) **syndrome due to stagnation of** *qi* **and** *blood*

Main Symptoms and Signs: Harder nodes in the penis which are painful because of overstrain; irritability, impatience, white tongue coating, and taut pulse.

Therapeutic Principles: Regulate *qi*, promote *blood* circulation, resolve phlegm and disperse nodes.

Recipe: *Huajian sanjie tang*

Radix Bupleuri	10 g
Rhizoma Cyperi	10 g
Thallus Laminariae seu Echloniae	20 g
Sargassum	20 g
Rhizoma Achyranthis Bidentatae	15 g
Radix Paeoniae Rubra	15 g
Rhizoma Sparganii	10 g
Rhizoma Curcumae	10 g
Bombyx Batryticatus	10 g
Rhizoma Pinelliae	10 g
Spina Gleditsiae	10 g
Semen Sinapis Album	10 g

All the above drugs are to be decocted in water for oral administration.

2) **syndrome due to** *yin* – **deficiency of the liver and kidney**

Main Symptoms and Signs: Nodes in the penis with slightly red skin and mild pain, soreness and weakness of the loins and legs, vertigo, slightly red tongue with little coating, and thready slightly rapid pulse.

Therapeutic Principles: Nourish yin, clear away heat, resolve phlegm and disperse nodes.

Recipe: *Liuwei dihuang tang*

Radix Rehmanniae Praeparata	30 g
Fructus Corni	12 g
Cortex Moutan Radicis	10 g
Rhizoma Alismatis	10 g
Poria	12 g
Rhizoma Dioscoreae	12 g
Rhizoma Achyranthis Bidentatae	12 g
Bombyx Batryticatus	10 g
Bulbus Fritillariae Thunbergii	10 g
Rhizoma Pinelliae	10 g
Cortex Phellodendri	6 g
Pericarpium Citri Reticulatae	10 g
Radix Glycyrrhizae	6 g

All the above drugs are to be decocted in water for oral administration.

Together with decoction, 5 – 10 tablets of *Sichong pian* (same amount of *Scolopendra*, *Scorpio*, *Lumbricus* and *Eupolyphaga seu Steleophaga*, ground into fine powder and made into tablets, each weighing 0.3 g.) or 6 – 8 tablets of *Sanjie pian* may be taken once daily.

Chapter Thirteen
Balanoposthitis

Balanoposthitis is the inflammation of both the balanus and prepuce due to reproduction of bacteria resulting from intracystic smegma and uncleanliness in redundant phimosis or prepuce. It is included in the category of *Gānchuāng* (chancre).

ETIOLOGY AND PATHOGENESIS

The penis is controlled by the liver and the anus and external genital organs are dominated by the kidney. During the acute stage, damp-heat in the *Liver Meridian* goes downwards to meet the damp-evil that invades the redundant prepuce in the external genitalia due to abrasion of the balanus and local uncleanliness, where they stay and turn into heat which spoils the tissue into pus. If fire due to long accumulation of damp-heat in the *Liver Meridian* goes downwards to burn the kidney-*yin*, there will appear syndrome due to *yin*-deficiency of the liver and kidney during the advanced stage.

MAIN SYMPTOMS AND SIGNS

Red swelling, dampness, erosion and even small superficial ulcer with cream-white purulent secretion on the tunica intima of the balanus and prepuce; swelling, fever and mild pain and itching of the prepuce; enlarged and tender inguinal lymph nodes in most cases; no general symptoms except for chills and fever in severe cases; yellow greasy tongue coating, and taut slippery rapid pulse. Improper treatment of the prolonged one may lead to cementation at the part of prepuce and balanus, incapability of the prepuce to be everted, stricture of external orifice of urethra and dysuria.

DIFFERENTIAL DIAGNOSIS

1. soft chancre

Soft chancre is one of the sexual diseases. The pathogenic bacterium is *Hemophilic streptobacillus*. Several days later after a dirty sexual intercourse, there appear red pimples usually on the balanus. Afterwards, they become pustules and ulcers. The ulcers are identified by great number, superficiality, indistinct border, obvious red-swelling, softness, foul necrotic secretion and megalgia. Meanwhile, there exist enlarged inguinal lymph nodes on both sides which tend to suppurate and fester, forming fish-mouth-like ulcers.

2. hard chancre

This disease is the early manifestation of aquired lues. The pathogenic bacterium is *Spirochaeta pallida*. The ulcers on the balanus are characterized by only one in number, distinct border, flat bottom, hardness of cartilage, no obvious red-swelling around, and no itching or pain. Although the inguinal lymph nodes on both sides develop, they do not tend to suppurate and fester.

DIFFERENTIATION AND TREATMENT OF COMMON SYNDROMES

1. External Treatment

1) the acute stage

(1) The affected part is fumigated and washed with hot decoction of *Jiedu xiyao*, 20 minutes each time, twice daily.

(2) The ulcer with pus is fumigated and washed with the above decoction and then dusted with *Xiao niuhuang san* and *Dahuang youshabu*. The following is the ingredients of *Niuhuang san*.

Recipe:

Calculus Bovis	0.3 g
Rhizoma Coptidis	10 g
Concha Haliotidis	3 g
Olibanum Praeparata	3 g

Myrrha Praeparata	3 g
Concha Ostreae	3 g
Os Draconis Fossilia	3 g
Fel Ursi	1.5 g

Ground into very fine powder for use.

2) the chronic stage

(1) After fumigated and washed with Manxing kuiyang xiyao, the affected part is covered with Shengji san and Shengji yuhonggao youshabu.

Recipe: Manxing kuiyang xiyao

Radix Ampelopsis	12 g
Radix Angelicae Sinensis	15 g
Radix Astragali seu Hedysari	15 g
Radix Angelicae Dahuricae	15 g
Folium Artemisiae Argyi	12 g
Radix Glycyrrhizae	12 g
Radix Paeoniae Rubra	9 g
Olibanum	9 g
Myrrha Praeparata	9 g
fresh pig's bone	30 g

The fresh pig's bone is decocted to get 300 ml decoction, and then the other drugs are decocted in the decoction for 30 minutes to get the latter decoction. The area of a sore is washed and fumed with the latter decoction while it is hot, then the formal changes of medicine is taken.

(2) When there has appeared fresh granulation on the surface of ulcer without pus and necrosis, dressing change only with Dahuang youshabu or Shengji yuhonggao youshabu is enough.

2. Internal Treatment

1) the acute stage

Main Symptoms and Signs: Swelling, pain, hot sensation and itching of the penis and balanus on which there are even ulceration and purulent secretion, chills and fever in severe cases, deep-colored urine, yellow greasy tongue coating, and taut slippery rapid pulse.

Therapeutic Principles: Clear away heat from the liver, promote diuresis and detoxicate.

Recipe: *Longdan xiegan tang jiajian*

Radix Gentianae	10 g
Radix Bupleuri	10 g
Radix Cyathulae	10 g
Cortex Phellodendri	10 g
Radix Paeoniae Rubra	10 g
Fructus Kochiae	10 g
Semen Plantaginis	10 g
Flos Lonicerae	30 g
Rhizoma Smilacis Glabrae	30 g
Caulis Clematidis Armandii	6 g
Radix Glycyrrhizae	6 g

All the above drugs are to be decocted in water for oral administration.

Modification: For mild cases, *Longdan xiegan wan* may be taken with warm boiled water, 6 g each time, twice to three times daily.

2) the chronic stage

Main Symptoms and Signs: Slow-growing purplish red granulation on the surface of ulcer, soreness and weakness of the loins and knees, vertigo, reddened tongue with little coating, and thready slightly rapid pulse, all of which are due to *yin*-deficiency of the liver and kidney; or fresh granulation on the surface of ulcer with little pyogenic secretion, but no general discomfort.

Therapeutic Principles: Nourish the liver and kidney for the former, and external treatment for the latter.

Liuwei dihuang wan or *Qiju dihuang wan* are applied.

Administration: 10 g is taken with warm boiled water each time, 3 times daily.

Chapter Fourteen
Enuresis

Enuresis refers to syndromes due to uncontrollable and spontaneous urination. Clinically, it falls into two kinds. One refers to frequent spontaneous urination with dribbling urine, the other spontaneous urination during sleep. The former is common in the aged, the latter in children.

ETIOLOGY AND PATHOGENESIS

Insufficiency and weakness of qi of the lung, spleen and kidney weaken the function of the urinary bladder in storing urine so that urination can not be controlled and enuresis results.

MAIN POINTS OF DIAGNOSIS

1. Clinical features are uncontrolled diurnal or nocturnal enuresis without dysuria.
2. Careful examination should be made on the life habit and mental status of the children to make sure if there are infections of the urinary tract or organic disorders.
3. In laboratory examinations, routine urine examination and culture may help to find out urinary tract infection. Roentgenography and pyelography may show recessive spinal bifida and other deformities of the urinary tract.

DIFFERENTIATION AND TREATMENT OF COMMON SYNDROMES

1. **failure of consolidation of the kidney** qi

Main Symptoms and Signs: Involuntary micturition during sleep with dreams, fluctuation in severity, frequent and profuse light colored urine, pallor, cold limbs, soreness and weakness of the loins and legs. Pale tongue with white and thin coating, deep, thready and forceless pulse.

Therapeutic Principles: Warm the kidney and arrest enuresis.

Recipe:

Radix Aconiti Praeparata	9 g
Cortex Cinnamomi	6 g
Radix Astragali seu Hedysari	15 g
Radix Codonopsis Pilosulae	30 g
Oötheca Mantidis	15 g
Semen Cuscutae	9 g
Fructus Psoraleae	15 g
Fructus Alpiniae Oxyphyllae	15 g
Fructus Rubi	15 g

All the above drugs are to be decocted in water for oral administration.

2. qi deficiency in the lung and spleen

Main Symptoms and Signs: Enuresis during sleeping, frquent and scanty urination, listlessness, shortness of breath, unwillingness to speak, poor appetite, loose stool, spontaneous perspiration. Pale tongue, thready pulse.

Therapeutic Principles: Invigorate the spleen and replenish qi to arrest enuresis.

Recipe:

Radix Ginseng	6 g
Radix Astragali seu Hedysari	15 g
Rhizoma Atractylodis Macrocephalae	12 g
Rhizoma Dioscoreae	15 g
Radix Angelicae Sinensis	12 g
Fructus Rubi	12 g
Fructus Alpiniae Oxyphyllae	12 g
Fructus Schisandrae	6 g
Rhizoma Cimicifugae	9 g
Radix Bupleuri	9 g

Radix Glycyrrhizae Praeparata	6 g

3. damp – heat stagnation in the bladder

Main Symptoms and Signs: Enuresis during sleeping, scanty urine with fish-stink odor and yellow color, flushed face, thirst, irritability, insomnia. Red tongue with yellow and greasy coating, slippery and rapid pulse.

Therapeutic Principles: Remove damp – heat from the bladder.

Recipe:

Fructus Gardeniae	9 g
Herba Lophatheri	9 g
Herba Dianthi	12 g
Radix Clematidis	6 g
Semen Plantaginis	12 g
Radix Scutellariae	9 g
Folium Pyrrosiae	12 g
Radix Glycyrrhizae	6 g
Radix Asteris	12 g

All the above drugs are to be decocted in water for oral administration.

4. damp – heat accumulated in the *Liver Meridian*

Main Symptoms and Signs: Enuresis during sleeping, scanty urine with fish-stink odor and yellow color, irascible temperament or feverish sensation in the palms and soles, nocturnal muttering and teeth grinding, flushed face and lips, thin and yellowish fur, and taut and smooth pulse.

Therapeutic Principles: Remove pathogenic damp – heat from the *Liver Meridian*

Recipe:

Radix Gentianae	3 g
Fructus Gardeniae	9 g
Caulis Clematidis Armandii	
Radix Bupleuri	6 g
Radix Angelicae Sinensis	9 g
Radix Scutellariae	9 g
Rhizoma Alismatis	9 g
Semen Plantaginis	9 g

Folium Pyrrosiae	9 g
Radix Glycyrrhizae Praeprata	3 g

All the above drugs are to be decocted in water for oral administration.

5. enuresis during sleep (deficiency – cold of the kidney)

Main Symptoms and Signs: Enuresis during sleep often with dreaminess, usually accompanied in severe cases by listlessness, chills, cold limbs, emaciation, general debilitation, pale tongue with white coating, and thready weak pulse.

Therapeutic Principles: Tonify the heart and spleen, warm the kidney to control urination.

Recipe:

Oötheca Mantidis	30 g
Fructus Rubi	30 g
Radix Codonopsis	9 g
Radix Astragali seu Hedysari	9 g
Poria cum Ligno Hospite	9 g
Fructus Psoraleae	9 g
Os Draconis Fossilia	15 g
Rhizoma Acori Tatarinowii	12 g
Radix Glycyrrhizae Praeparata	6 g

All the above drugs are to be decocted in water for oral administration.

Recipe 2:

Oötheca Mantidis	
Semen Cuscutae	9 g
Fructus Alpiniae Oxyphyllae	15 g
Fructus Psoraleae	15 g
Fructus Rubi	15 g
Radix Aconiti Praeparata	6 g
Cortex Cinnamomi	4.5 g
Radix Astragali seu Hedysari	15 g
Radix Codonopsis Pilosulae	15 g

All the above drugs are to be decocted in water for oral administration.

Acupuncture and Moxibustion

1. body acupuncture

Main Points: Shènshū(BL23), Pángguāngshū(BL28), Zhōngjí(RN3), Sānyīnjiāo (SP6), and Dàdūn(LR1).

Complementary Points: Add Shénmén(HT7) for enuresis with dreams; add Píshū(BL20) and Zúsānlǐ(ST36) for loss of appetite.

Method: Use filiform needles to puncture the points with tonification and moxibustion.

2. scalp acupuncture

Prescription Points: *foot motor sensory area* and *reproduction area*..

Method: Puncture the areas along the skin. Twirl the needles for one minute. Electrotherapy is also applicable. Retain the needles for 15 minutes.

Massage

Press-knead Píshū(BL20) and Shènshū(BL23) 30 times each, scrub Yāoyǎn (EX-B7) 30 times, scrub horizontally the lumbosacral portion till it gets hot, knead Qìhǎi(RN6) and Guānyuán(RN4) 30 times each, strike digitally Zhōngjí (RN3) 30 times, rub *Dantian* clockwise and counterclockwise 30 times respectively, and scrub-knead Hégǔ(LI4), Zúsānlǐ(ST36) and Sānyīnjiāo(SP6) 30 times each.

Patients with dripping urination accompanied with dizziness, soreness of the loins and cold extremities should be treated by pressing-kneading Mìngmén(DU4) and Zhìshì(BL52) 30 times each and kneading Bǎihuì(DU20), Fēngchí(GB20), Qūchí(LI11) and Tàixī(KI3) 30 times each.

Patients with sallow complexion, mental fatigue and weakness, poor appetite and loose stool should be treated by pressing-kneading Wèishū(BL21) 30 times respectively, scrubbing the lower abdomen 30 times and pressing-kneading Chángqiáng(DU1) and Nèiguān(PC6) 30 times each.

Medicated Diet

1. Parch 9 g of *Fructus Alpiniae Oxyphyllae* with vinegar and grind it into fine

powder. Take it in 3 portions infused with boiled water for 6 to 7 days successively.

2. Clean one pig's bladder and parch it until it is done. Chew it slowly before swallowing it, or take it with a bit of wine.

3. Have a yellow hen and remove its feathers and internal organs, and cook it with *Radix Astragali seu Hedysari* 30 g and *Radix Rehmanniae Praeparata* 15 g until it is thoroughly done; take away the dregs and chicken bones. Add polished *round-grained rice* 120 g to cook gruel. Take it at will after seasoning it.

4. Make soup with 250 g to 500 g of dog meat and 20 g of *Semen Sojae Nigrum*. Finish it as a dose in two portions in one day. Take one every other day. Take 5 to 6 doses in all.

5. Recipe:

pork urinary bladder	1
Flos Sophorae	15 g
Radix Codonopsis Pilosulae	15 g

Have the pork urinary bladder cut open, washed clean and cut into cubes, and *Flos Sophorae* and *Radix Codonopsis Pilosulae* wrapped up with a piece of cloth; then put them into a pot and add water to cook them until the bladder is thoroughly done; remove the residues and take it after it has been seasoned.

Take one dose every other day and take seven to eight doses in all. This recipe is applicable to the disease caused by deficiency of both the spleen-qi and lung-qi.

Recipe:

Fructus Mume	6 g
Coccum Bombycis	20 g
Fructus Ziziphi Jujubae	10
white sugar	50 g

Make decoction for oral administration with the above ingredients

Take it before 4 o'clock p.m. every day, and that for days successively. it is applicable to the children who have the diseases of the type with deficiency of the kidney-qi.

Qigong

Assume the standing posture. Clench both hands into fists to support the lumbar soft tissues on both sides of the body. Take the waist as an axis and turn leftwards for 6 circles. Then turn rightwards for 6 circles. Assume the standing or sitting posture. Rub the bilateral lumbar sides with both hands up and down for 36 times, with the mind on the lumbar region. Hold the scrotum with the right hand and press flatly the pubes under the junction of the pubic bones with the left hand. Two hands hold and press the scrotum simultaneously for 81 times. Then the hands are changed to hold and press the scrotum 81 times.

Chapter Fifteen
Diabetes Insipidus

Diabetes Insipidus is caused by hyposecretion of antidiuretic hormone resulting from hypothalamus-pituitary lesion. It can also be secondary to other diseases. The state of illness may be mild or severe, transient or permanent. The disease belongs to the category of "Xiāokě" in traditional Chinese medicine.

MAIN POINTS OF DIAGNOSIS

1. Polyuria, polydipsia and increased water intake are the principal features. If water intake is restricted, severe dehydration may occur.

2. The etiology of primary diabetes insipidus remains indeterminate. Secondary cases may be initiated by tumor, infection or trauma of the hypothalamus-pituitary system or the adjacent tissues. There they have the corresponding histories and clinical symptoms and signs.

3. **accessory examinations**

1) The specific gravity of urine is reduced and usually less than 1.006. The osmotic pressure of urine is also reduced.

2) The osmotic pressure of plasma is elevated. There may appear dizziness, dysphoria, tachycardia or disorder of consciousness, the so-called hyperosmotic syndrome.

3) Water-deprivation test and hypertonic saline test are used to distinguish diabetes insipidus from psychogenic polydipsia and polyuria. Water-deprivation test is dangerous, and now is rarely performed.

DIFFERENTIATION AND TREATMENT OF COMMON SYNDROMES

Deficiency of the Kidney - *qi*

Main Symptoms and Signs: Polydipsia, frequent and profuse urination, emaciation, aching pain in the lumbus, lassitude. The case exhibiting more symptoms and signs of deficiency of the kidney - *yin* is marked as feverish sensation in the palms and soles, restlessness, red tongue with little fur, deep, thready and rapid pulse; while the case presenting more symptoms and signs of deficiency of the kidney - *yang* is manifested as light color urine, aversion to cold, impotence, pale tongue with whitish fur, and deep, thready and weak pulse.

Therapeutic Principles: Invigorate the kidney and arrest polyuria.

Recipe: *Liuwei dihuang wan jiajian*

Radix Rehmanniae Praeparata	15 g
Fructus Corni	15 g
Rhizoma Dioscoreae	15 g
Fructus Lycii	15 g
Semen Cuscutae	12 g
Radix Ophiopogonis	15 g
Oötheca Mantidis	20 g
Fructus Schisandrae	10 g
Radix Glycyrrhizae	15 g

All the above drugs are to be decocted in water for oral administration.

Modification: In addition to the above recipe, for treating those presenting more symptoms and signs of deficiency of the kidney - *yin*, 15 grams of *Radix Rehmanniae*, 12 grams of *Radix Scutellariae*, 18 grams of *Radix Trichosanthis* and 10 grams of *Galla Sinensis* should be added. For treating those exhibiting more symptoms and signs of deficiency of the kidney - *yang*, the following ingredients are added: *Radix Aconiti Praeparata* 10 g, *Cortex Cinnamomi* 6 g, *Fructus Psoraleae* 12 g, *Fructus Alpiniae Oxyphyllae* 10 g, *Fructus Rubi* 12 g, *Radix Astragali seu Hedysari* 15 g.

Chapter Sixteen
Retention of Urine

Retention of urine refers to difficulty in urination resulting in large amount of urine accumulated in the bladder, clinically characterized by blockage of urine and distention and fullness in the lower abdomen. In traditional Chinese medicine, it belongs to the category of "Wuniao".

DIFFERENTIATION AND TREATMENT OF COMMON SYNDROMES

1. **accumulation of damp – heat in the bladder**

Main Symptoms and Signs: Scanty, hot and deep – colored urine or retention of urine, distention and fullness of the lower abdomen, bitter and sticky taste in the mouth, thirst but without any desire to drink, constipation. Red tongue with yellow and greasy coating, rapid pulse.

Therapeutic Principles: Clear away heat and purge fire, induce diuresis for treating retention of urine.

Recipe:

Talcum	30 g
Radix Glycyrrhizae	15 g
Fructus Gardeniae	18 g
Caulis Akebiae	15 g
Semen Plantaginis (decocted after being wrapped in a piece of cloth)	
Radix Asteris	15 g
Herba Dianthi	15 g
Radix et Rhizoma Rhei	9 g

2. collapse of the central *qi*

Main Symptoms and Signs: Dribbling urination or retention of urine, distention and dropping pain in the lower abdomen, lassitude and shortness of breath, loss of appetite. Pale tongue with thin coating, deep and weak pulse.

Therapeutic Principles: Send up the clear and send down the turbidity.

Recipe:

Radix Astragali seu Hedysari	15 g
Radix Ginseng	9 g
Radix Glycyrrhizae	9 g
Radix Angelicae Sinensis	9 g
Pericarpium Citri Reticulatae	9 g
Rhizoma Cimicifugae	6 g
Radix Bupleuri	6 g
Rhizoma Atractylodis Macrocephalae	9 g
Cortex Cinnamomi	6 g
Medulla Tetrapanacis	9 g
Semen Plantaginis (decocted after being wrapped in a piece of cloth)	9 g

3. decline of life gate fire

Main Symptoms and Signs: Dribbling urination or retention of urine, pallor, listlessness, chillness below the lumbus, soreness and weakness of the loins and knees. Pale tongue, deep and thready pulse, weak pulse at the *chi* region.

Therapeutic Principles: Warm and reinforce the kidney *yang*, produce *qi* and induce diuresis.

Recipe:

Radix Aconiti Praeparata	15 g
Cortex Cinnamomi	9 g
Radix Rehmanniae Praeparata	30 g
Fructus Corni	15 g
Rhizoma Dioscoreae	15 g
Poria	15 g
Cortex Moutan Radicis	9 g
Rhizoma Alismatis	15 g

| *Rhizoma Achyranthis Bidentatae* | 18 g |

Semen Plantaginis

(decocted after being wrapped in a piece of cloth)   9 g

Acupuncture and Moxibustion

Main Points: **Zhōngjí(RN3)**, and **Sānyīnjiāo(SP6)**.

Complementary Points: Add **Pángguāngshū(BL28)** and **Wěiyáng(BL39)** for the accumulation of damp－heat in the bladder; **Shuǐdào(ST28)** and **Shuǐquán(KI5)** for the collapse of the central qi; **Mìngmén(DU4)**, **Shènshū(BL23)**, **Bǎihuì(DU20)**, **Guānyuán(RN4)** and **Yángchí(SJ4)** for the decline of the life gate fire.

Method: Use filiform needles to puncture the points with sedation for the excessive type, and with tonification and moxibustion for the deficient type.

Massage

1. Push **Jīmén(SP11)**, press－knead *dantian* and **Sānyīnjiāo(SP6)**. The massage is performed once a day. In severe cases, it is done twice a day or repeatedly until urination happens. If there is no effect, the duration of manipulation can be prolonged or some other therapies may be taken.

Modification: For downward flow of damp－heat, add clearing *xiaochang*, kneading *xiaotianxin* and reducing *liufu*.

For deficiency of the kidney－*yang*, reinforce *shenjing*, knead *erma*, push *sanguan*, and knead **Shènshū(BL23)** can be added. Apart from the manipulations mentioned above, clearing *dachang* and pushing－down *qijiegu* can be added for patients with constipation.

2. Rub the lower abdomen in clockwise direction for 6 minutes; press and knead **Zhōngjí(RN3)**, **Qìhǎi(RN6)**, **Guānyuán(RN4)**, **Sānyīnjiāo(SP6)**, **Yīnlíngquán(SP9)**, **Pángguāngshū(BL28)**, **Shènshū(BL23)** and **Mìngmén(DU4)** for one minute respectively; rub and knead **Bìguān(ST31)** and **Zúwǔlǐ(LR10)** for 6 minutes till the sore and distending sensation appears; chafe horizontally the *Bladder Meridian*, **Shènshū(BL23)** and **Mìngmén(DU4)** till the heat penetrates.

Retention of Urine

Qigong

1. First apply both palms to push and rub the sacral region up and down 300 times. Then overlap the palms on the abdomen. Knead and rub the abdomen from the right to the left in exhalation. Meanwhile, relax the anus and the abdomen; slightly draw in the abdomen and stop both palms temporarily in inhalation. Do for 14 or 28 breaths altogether.

2. Assume the standing or sitting posture. Place the right palms flat on the lower abdomen; inhale slowly, and utter "Chuī" in exhalation. Rub the lower abdomen gently with the right palm. Do for 10 or 20 breaths. The method is applicable to the accumulation of damp-heat in the bladder.

3. Assume the standing posture with the feet apart in the shoulder width. Stand in a relaxed and tranquil state; regulate the breathing evenly; get rid of the distracting thoughts and face to the sun. When the sun rises from the horizon, slightly droop the eyelids, but still able to see the soft and slight red sunlight; inhale the *qi* of the sunlight essence through the nose, and breathe in one mouthful of it (imagine this in the mind). Hold the breath and concentrate the mind; swallow it slowly along with the exhalation and send it down to *Dantian*. Repeat this procedure for 10 times. Then naturally relax and tranquilize, concentrate the mind peacefully for a short while and then naturally limber up the body for a moment before finishing the exercises. The maneuver is good for the decline of the life gate fire.

Chapter Seventeen
Chyluria

Chyluria is usually due to bancroftosis but occasionally due to tuberculosis of urinary system or tumors. Its main clinical manifestations are intermittent recurrence of cream – white urine, hematuria in most patients, swelling of testicle, hydrocele of tunica vaginalis of scrotum, elephantiasis crus, etc., and microfilaria of blood filaria possibly found in blood examination done in the night. It is named in traditional Chinese medicine "turbid urine" according to the color of urine.

ETIOLOGY AND PATHOGENESIS

This disease is caused by downward flow of damp – heat due to over – intake of fatty and sweet food or by downward flow of refined nutritious substances due to exhaustion of *qi* and *blood* resulting from deficiency of the spleen and due to failure to astringe resulting from deficiency of the kidney.

DIFFERENTIATION AND TREATMENT OF COMMON SYNDROMES

During the early stage, this disease is mainly due to downward flow of damp – heat. So, the treatment should be conducted mainly by clearing away heat and inducing diuresis. When it becomes protracted and recurrent, the spleen and kidney have been made weak. At this time, the treatment should be, accordingly, concentrated on invigorating the spleen – *qi* and reinforcing the kidney. Simultaneously, the symptoms and cause should be treated together.

1. **type of downward flow of damp – heat**
Main Symptoms and Signs: Turbid and cream – white urine sometimes with

coagula which becomes evident whenever fish or meat is eaten, no pain during urinating, full and choking sensation in the chest and epigastrium, thirst without desire for drinking, yellow thick greasy tongue coating, and soft rapid pulse.

Therapeutic Principles: Eliminate damp-heat.

Recipe: *Ruminiao tang*

Rhizoma Dioscoreae Hypoglaucae	30 g
Spora Lygodii	30 g
Folium Pyrrosiae	30 g
Poria	12 g
Radix Rehmanniae	15 g
Herba Polygoni Avicularis	15 g
Fructus Ligustri Lucidi	12 g
Flos Carthami	9 g
Cortex Phellodendri	6 g

Modification: In case of lassitude, poor appetite and edema, the drugs added are *Radix Codonopsis Pilosulae* 15 g, *Rhizoma Atractylodis Macrocephalae* 15 g, *Semen Euryales* 30 g.

In case of hematuria, the drugs added are *Rhizoma Imperatae* 30 g, *Herba Leonuri* 30 g, *Herba Agrimoniae* 15 g and *Petiolus Trachycarpi Carbonisatus* 9 g.

In case of slow loss of protein, the drugs added are *Semen Nelumbinis* 30 g, *Fructus Rosae Laevigatae* 15 g, *Rhizoma Atractylodis Macrocephalae* 15 g and *Semen Cuscutae* 15 g.

In case of lumbago, the drugs added are *Herba Taraxaci* 30 g, *Rhizoma Cibotii* 15 g and *Radix Dipsaci* 15 g.

2. type of failure of the deficient kidney to perform its astringing function

Main Symptoms and Signs: Turbid urine, restlessness, fever, thirst, soreness and weakness of the loins and knees, fatigue, acratia, dizziness, blurred vision, reddened tongue with little coating, and deep thready or thready rapid pulse.

Therapeutic Principles: Reinforce the kidney for consolidation.

Recipe: *Liuwei dihuang tang* and *Tusizi wan*

Radix Rehmanniae Praeparata	30 g
Fructus Corni	12 g
Rhizoma Dioscoreae	15 g
Semen Cuscutae	24 g
Fructus Lycii	15 g

Semen Nelumbinis	12 g
Semen Euryales	15 g
Os Draconis Fossilia	30 g
Concha Ostreae	30 g
Fructus Schisandrae	9 g

Modification: In case of severe lumbago, the drugs added are *Radix Dipsaci* 15 g, *Cortex Eucommiae* 15 g, *Rhizoma Cimicifugae* 12 g.

In case of remarkable deficiency of the spleen, the drugs added are *Radix Codonopsis Pilosulae* 15 g, *Rhizoma Atractylodis Macrocephalae* 12 g and *Radix Astragali seu Hedysari* 15 g.

In case of deficiency and weakness of kidney – *yang* marked by cold limbs, loose stools, pale tongue with white coating, and deep weak pulse, the drugs added are *Cornu Cervi Pantotrichum* 9 g, *Fructus Psoraleae* 12 g, *Radix Aconiti Lateralis Praeparata* 9 g and *Cortex Cinnamomi* 6 g.

3. type of downward flow of the spleen – *qi*

Main Symptoms and Signs: Turbid urine which becomes more evident due to overstrain, sallow complexion, lassitude, weakness, pale tongue with thin white coating, and weak pulse.

Therapeutic Principles: Supplement *qi* to send up the lucid *yang*.

Recipe: *Buzhong yiqi tang*

Radix Astragali seu Hedysari	15 g
Radix Codonopsis	12 g
Rhizoma Atractylodis Macrocephalae	12 g
Radix Angelicae Sinensis	9 g
Pericarpium Citri Reticulatae	9 g
Rhizoma Cimicifugae	6 g
Radix Bupleuri	6 g
Radix Glycyrrhizae Praeparata	6 g
Fructus Jujubae	5 dates

All the above drugs are to be decocted in water for oral administration.

Modification: In case of poor appetite, abdominal distention, emaciation and insufficiency of *qi* of the middle – *jiao*, the drugs added are *Rhizoma Dioscoreae* 15 g, *Semen Euryales* 12 g, *Fructus Ginkgo* 9 g.

Prevention

1. Patients with chyluria should avoid overstrain and heavy food.
2. Cure bancroftosis.

Chapter Eighteen
Impotence

Impotence is mostly due to sexual neurasthenia, with clinical manifestations of no or poor erection of penis and interference of normal sexual life.

DIFFERENTIATION AND TREATMENT OF COMMON SYNDROMES

Downward flow of the damp heat, softness and relaxation of penis, the deficiency at the anterior, the excess at the posterior altogether result in impotence.

1. **decline of the fire of vital gate**

Fire decline off the vital gate, consumption of essence and qi, decline of the kidney *yang*, impotence as the result.

Main Symptoms and Signs: Debility of penis erection, thin semina, dilute and cold, pallor of face, dizziness and tinnitus, soreness and weakness of loin and knees. Aversion to cold and cold limbs, listlessness, malaise, amnesia, dreaminess. Pale tongue with thin white proper. Deep fine and weak pulse.

Therapeutic Principles: Reinforce the vital gate using drugs with warm or hot property; replenish the semina and promote erection.

Recipe:

Radix Rehmanniae Praeparata	12 g
Radix Polygoni Multiflori Praeparata	15 g
Fructus Corni	12 g
Rhizoma Dioscoreae	12 g
Radix Mori	12 g
Herba Epimedii	12 g
Fructus Lycii	15 g
Cornu Cervi Pantotrichum	10 g

Herba Ephedrae Praparatum	8 g
Rhizoma Acori Graminei	
Radix Polygalae	10 g

All the above drugs are to be decocted in water for oral administration.

Modification: For prominent *qi* deficiency, add *Radix Ginseng* and *Radix Astragali seu Hedysari*; for deficiency of heart *qi*, amnesia, and dreaminess, add *Radix Panacis Quinquefolii*, *Fructus Schisandrae* and *Semen Biotae*.

Moxibustion: **Shènshū (BL23), Mìngmén (DU4), Guānyuán (RN4), Cìliáo (BL32).**

2. downward flow of damp-heat

Damp-heat in the lower *jiao*, where *yang qi* can not reach, penis flabby and soft.

Main Symptoms and Signs: Flabby and soft penis, wet and foul scrotum, heaviness of body, especially the lower limbs, deep-colored urine. Sticky and foul mouth. Yellow and slimy tongue fur, weak and rapid pulse.

Therapeutic Principles: Clear the heat and remove dampness with diuresis, strengthen *yang* and treat impotence.

Recipe: *Sanmiao san jiajian*

Cortex Phellodendri	10 g
Rhizoma Atractylodis	12 g
Radix Gentianae	12 g
Fructus Gardeniae	10 g
Rhizoma Alismatis	21 g
Rhizoma Achyranthis Bidentatae	12 g
Semen Plantaginis (decocted after being wrapped in a piece of cloth)	15 g
Radix Angelicae Sinensis	12 g
Radix Rehmanniae	15 g
Herba Ephedrae Praeparatum	6 g

All the above drugs are to be decocted in water for oral administration.

Modification: *Yin* damage by damp heat, thirsty with preference to drinks, add *Rhizoma Dioscoreae*; exuberance of heat evil, omit *Herba Ephedrae*, add *Gypsum Fibrosum* and *Radix Scutellariae*.

3. deficiency of the kidney *yang*

Main Symptoms and Signs: Failure of the penis in erection or weak erection, accompanied by dizziness, tinnitus, soreness and weakness of the back and knees, chills in the four extremities. Pale tongue with white coating, deep, slow and weak pulse.

Therapeutic Principles: Replenish the kidney and strengthen *yang*

Recipe:

Herba Epimedii	12 g
Fructus Psoraleae	12 g
Herba Cistanchis	15 g
Plastrum Testudinis	12 g
Radix Rehmanniae Praeparata	20 g
Cortex Cinnamomi	6 g
Pericarpium Citri Reticulatae	9 g

4. blood deficiency of the heart and spleen

Main Symptoms and Signs: Failure of the penis in erection or weak erection, accompanied by palpitation, shortness of breath, lassitude, sallow complexion, poor appetite. Pale tongue, thready and weak pulse.

Therapeutic Principles: Nourish the heart and replenish the spleen.

Recipe:

Radix Angelicae Sinensis	12 g
Radix Rehmanniae Praeparata	15 g
Radix Paeoniae Alba	15 g
Radix Ophiopogonis	12 g
Rhizoma Polygonati	9 g
Radix Scutellariae	12 g
Radix Asparagi	12 g
Radix Polygoni Multiflori	15 g

239 cases were treated with the above methods. Among which there are 96 ases with mental impotence, 89 cases with impotence caused by chronic prostatitis, 9 cases due to agenesis of sex gland, 45 cases with impotence suspected to be organic. As a result, 52 cases were cured; 68 showed considerable improvement; 99 cases partially improved. The total effective rate was 91.7%. It was found

Impotence

through observation that the above methods listed most effective in treating cases of mental impotence, less effective with cases of impotence caused by prostatitis and least effective on impotence due to agenesis of sex gland. The results of treatment were better for cases with sick course within 3 years. No effect was achieved for cases with sick course over 10 years.

6. wine for tonifying *yang* and benefiting kidney
Recipe:

Gecko	a pair
Hippocampus	10 g
Cornu Cervi Pantotrichum	10 g
Radix Ginseng Rubra	15 g
Fructus Lycii	50 g
Herba Epimedii	30 g
Fructus Schisandrae	30 g

Administration: After the above drugs are cleanly washed, they are soaked in 2.5 kg of white wine for 7 days. 35 g of the spirits is taken before sleep every night. 2 months consisted of one course.

107 cases ere treated with the above method. 54 of them were almost cured after one course of treatment; 35 cases showed considerable improvement after 2 courses of treatment. The total effective rate was 83.2%.

Acupuncture and Moxibustion

Point: **Juyang** (at the median of the linking line between **Zhìbiān**(BL54) and **Huántiào**(GB30), the needle is inserted obliquely and directed to opposite symphysis until the patient felt a sensation of numbness, distention and pain at the base of his penis.

Modification: For insufficient *yang* in the kidney, **Guānyuán**(RN4), **Mìngmén**(DU4), **Shènshū**(BL23), **Sānyīnjiāo**(SP6) are punctured additionally, and **Shènshū**(BL23), **Mìngmén**(DU4) are applied with moxibustion; for deficiency in both the spleen and heart, **Xīnshū**(BL15), **Nèiguān**(PC6), **Zhōngwǎn**(RN12), **Zúsānlǐ**(ST36), **Píshū**(BL20), **Guānyuán**(RN4), **Sānyīnjiāo**(SP6) and **Shènshū**(BL23) are added; for *yin* deficiency in the heart and kidney, **Zhōngjí**(RN3), **Cìliáo**(BL32), **Sānyīnjiāo**(SP6), **Dàlíng**(PC7), **Shénmén**(HT7) and **Fùliū**(KI7) are added.

Manipulation: Normal methods of tonification and attenuation are used at the point **Juyang**. Single attenuation method is used at **Dàlíng(PC7)** and single tonification of lifting, thrusting, twisting and twirling at other selected points. The needling sensation at points **Guānyuán(RN4)** and **Zhōngjí(RN3)** is required to reach glans penis. The needles are retained in the points for 30 minutes. The acupuncture is applied once every other day. 12 times consisted of one treatment. An interval of one week between two courses is required.

258 cases were treated with the above method. 87 cases were cured; 157 cases improved. The curative rate was 33.72%; the effective rate was 94.57%.

MASSAGE

Manipulation:
1) **transverse rubbing of the lower abdomen**

The patient is to lie in a supine position; masseur placed his palms on both sides of the patient's umbilicus at the interior margin of ilium and rubbed the region horizontally towards the center of the abdomen for 5 – 10 minutes.

2) **kneading point Mìngmén(DU4)**

The doctor uses the dorsal part of the index finger or thenar to knead the point **Mìngmén(DU4)** in prone position for 5 – 10 minutes.

3) **pushing waist with fingers**

The patient is to lie in prone position. The doctor places his thumbs on the patient's **Shènshū(BL23)** and his other fingers on the waist region. Then pushing method is performed from the interior to the margin of anterior ribs in an exterior – inferior direction for 5 – 10 minutes.

4) Pressing **Sānyīnjiāo(SP6)** for 5 – 10 minutes.

5) Press **Zúsānlǐ(ST36)** for 5 – 10 minutes.

All the above maneuvers are performed once a day. 7 days consisted of one course of treatment. An interval of 3 – 5 days between two courses is required.

20 cases were treated with the above method. 12 cases recovered completely; 5 cases improved.

Qigong

1. Twist the spermatic cord with fingers

Assume the sitting posture. Symmetrize the forefingers, middle fingers and thumbs of the two hands respectively. Hold up the spermatic cord on both sides of the root of the penis with the fingers and twist left and right for 50 times respectively. Relax the whole body. Breathe naturally and pay attention to the induction produced by twisting the spermatic cords with the two hands until there is a slight sore and distending sensation.

2. Knead the testicles

Assume the sitting posture. Use the right hand to clasp the scrotum and penis together with the part of the hand between the thumb and forefinger facing forward, leaving the scrotum and testicles outside the part between the thumb and forefinger, and grasp the root portion of the scrotum and testicles tightly. First press the hollow of the left palm on the testicle on the left side and knead it 50 times. Then change the hands and knead the testicle on the right side in the same way for 50 times. Breathe naturally and focus the mind on the hollow of the palm which is kneading the testicle.

3. Rub – roll the testicles between the fingers

Assume the sitting posture. Use the palmar sides of the forefinger and middle finger of each hand to prop up the inferior part of the testicle on the identical side respectively. Then press the thumbs on the testicles respectively and rub them between the fingers left and right 50 times respectively.

4. Jack the testicles

Assume the sitting posture. use the palmar sides of the forefinger and middle finger of each hand to prop up the testicle on the identical side respectively. Then use the tips of the fingers to jack up the testicles toward the directions of the groins and then drop down. Do 3 times altogether. Inhale slowly when jacking up and exhale slowly when dropping down. It will be enough when the location of the groins has a slightly expanding and distending sensation. Do not exert too much pressure.

The above four sections have the functions of promoting the formation of sperms and the secretion of male sex hormone. They are important maneuvers to strengthen the fire of vital gate and thus reinforce the kidney *yang* and replenish the essence *qi*.

Medicated Diet

1. Boil 250 g of *mutton* and cut it into slices after it is done. Then mix well with 15 g of pounded *garlic*, proportional amount of *cooked oil*, *capsicum fruit*, *soy sauce* and *table salt* for eating.

2. Stir-fry 120 g of *chive* and 200 g of fresh *river shrimps* in cooking oil and with right amount of table salt for eating.

Recipe: *Sea Cucumber and Mutton Soup*

Stichopus Japonicus	250 g
mutton	250 g
Rhizoma Zingiberis Recens	
table salt	

Stew the first two ingredients together. Season it with fresh *ginger* and *table salt* before it is eaten.

Recipe: *Gecko and Psoralea Fruit Powder*

Gecko	a pair
Fructus Psoraleae	25 g
spirits	

Stir-fry the *geckoes* in spirits and dry them over a fire, and then grind the *geckoes* and *Fructus Psoraleae* into fine powder. To be taken with warm spirits, 1.5 g each time.

Recipe: *Xianlingpi jiu*

Herba Epimedii	60 g
plain spirits	500 ml

Fill a gauze bag with *Herba Epimedii*, soak it in *plain spirits* and seal the container. It can be taken after it has been soaked for three days. To be taken before sleep, 10 to 15 ml each time.

All the recipes above can reinforce the kidney and strengthen *yang*. Patients with impotence can choose one or two from among them regular eating according to the state of their illness.

Chapter Nineteen
Male Sterility

Male Sterility (MS) means infertility caused by disorders of male reproductive system. its clinical manifestations include abnormal sperm such as spermacrasia, aspermia, dead spermatozoon, azoospermia, etc., and disturbance of sexual function such as impotence, spermatorrhea, non — ejaculation etc.. The cause of the disease is rather complex, it may be roughly classified into two categories: the functional cause and the organic one or the primary one and secondary one. In traditional Chinese medicine, male sterility belongs to the categories of "*cold semen*", "*scanty semen*", "*impotence*" and "*persistent erection*" etc..

DIFFERENTIATION AND TREATMENT OF COMMON SYNDROMES

1. Deficit due to deficiency of kidney

Main Symptoms and Signs: Lumbago, weak legs, fatigue, lack of strength, clear urine in larger quantities, much urine at night, indifferent sexual desire, long — time infertility after marriage, pale tongue with thin — white coating, slender and taut or slender — soft and forceless pulse.

Recipe:

Radix Rehmanniae Praeparata	15 g
Rhizoma Dioscoreae	15 g
Radix Polygoni Multiflori	15 g
Fructus Mori	15 g
Radix Astragali seu Hedysari	15 g
Semen Plantaginis	12 g
Fructus Lycii	12 g
Semen Cuscutae	12 g
Fructus Rubi	12 g

Fructus Corni   6 g

Modification: For cases with emphasis on *yang* deficiency, *Herba Epimedii*, *Rhizoma Curculiginis* at 15 g each, *Radix Morindae Officinalis* 10 g, *Colla Cornus Cervi* 12 g are added; for cases with emphasis on *yin* deficiency, *Fructus Ligustri Lucidi*, *Herba Ecliptae* at 12 g each, *Colla Plastri Testudinis* 15 g are added; for spermacrasia, *Colla Plastri Testudinis* and *Colla Cornus Cervi* (both melted) are swallowed at 5 g each with honey and egg; for cases having much monstrous sperm, *Radix Angelicae Sinensis*, *Semen Persicae* at 10 g each, and *Radix Salviae Miltiorrhizae* 15 g are added; for spermatorrhea, *Oötheca Mantidis* 10 g, *Semen Euryales* 15 g, *Fructus Rosae Laevigatae* 15 g, *Rhizoma Alismatis* 12 g, *Cortex Phellodendri* 10 g are added; for azoospermia, *Radix Codonopsis Pilosulae* 15 g, *Radix Angelicae Sinensis* 10 g, *Colla Corii Asini* 10 g and *Radix Astragali seu Hedysari* 15 g are added.

2. Damp-heat in lower-*jiao*

Main Symptoms and Signs: Swelling and cramps in the perineum and lower abdomen, thirst, bitter taste in mouth, yellowish urine, red tongue with yellow-greasy coating, string-like and slippery pulse.

Recipe:

Radix Rehmanniae	15 g
Rhizoma Polygoni Cuspidati	6 g
Flos Lonicerae	15 g
Herba Dianthi	12 g
Semen Plantaginis	12 g
Rhizoma Dioscoreae Septemlobae	10 g
Cortex Phellodendri	10 g
Caulis Akebiae	10 g
Talcum	30 g
Radix Glycyrrhizae	5 g

Modification: For dysphoria and insomnia, *Fructus Gardeniae* 10 g, *Caulis Polygoni Multiflori* 15 g, *Cortex Albiziae* 10 g are added; for purulent sperm, *Herba Taraxaci* 15 g, *Rhizoma Smilacis Glabrae* 15 g are added; for dribbling urine, *Herba Leonuri*, *Fructus Alpiniae Oxyphyllae* at 12 g each are added; for abnormal seminal liquefaction, *Radix Salviae Miltiorrhizae* 15 g, *Radix Paeoniae Rubra* 12 g, *Rhizoma Acori Graminei* 6 g, *Radix Polygalae* 5 g are added; for non-ejaculation during coitus, *Squama Manitis* 10 g, *Nidus Vespae* 10 g (burned to ash and taken with the decoction), *Fructus Liquidambaris* 10 g are added.

Administration: All the above drugs are to be decocted in water for oral administration. One month consisted of one course of treatment. For patients with prostatitis, the third decoction from the above formula is used for a 20 - minute of hip bath before bed time at the same time of oral intake.

78 cases were treated with the above prescription. Of them, 50 cases, that is, 64% of the cases belonged to the type "deficit due to deficiency in the kidney"; 28 cases or 36% of the cases were grouped into the type "dampness - heat of lower - *jiao*". But statistically, no distinctive difference was found between the two types. it was found through observation that in the five cases who had no response, 3 cases had aspermia. This shows that one confronts definite difficulties in treating aspermia with the aid of traditional Chinese medicine.

Simple Recipes and Proved Recipes

1. infertility of abnormal sperm with semen - benefiting decoction

Recipe:

Radix Rehmanniae Praeparata	15 g
Herba Epimedii	15 g
Radix Codonopsis Pilosulae	15 g
Rhizoma Curculiginis	10 g
Semen Cuscutae	10 g
Fructus Rubi	10 g
Fructus Mori	10 g
Radix Angelicae Sinensis	10 g
Fructus Corni	10 g
Radix Astragali seu Hedysari	10 g
Radix Dipsaci	10 g
Semen Astragali Complanati	10 g
Poria	10 g
Peni et Testes Callorhini	1/2 piece

Modification: In case of leukocytes in the seminal fluid showing damp - heat in lower - *jiao*, *Rhizoma Smilacis Glabrae* 30 g, *Herba Lophatheri* 10 g, *Flos Lonicerae* 20 g are added; in case of spermatorrhea and premature ejaculation,

Herba Cynomorii, *Fructus Schisandrae* at 10 g each, *Semen Euryales* 15 g are added.

All the above drugs are to be decocted in water for oral administration. To be taken twice a day, in the morning and in the evening respectively. Half a month consisted of one course of treatment.

97 cases were treated with the above method. 69 cases were clinically cured, accounting for 70.1%; 22 cases improved, accounting for 22.7%. The total effective rate was 92.8%. The shortest time of treatment was 15 days and the longest 60 days. The spouses of 46 cases conceived after treatment, accounting for 47.4%. This group of cases included spermacrasia, incomplete liquifying of seminal fluid, azoospermia, monstrous sperm, aspermia and dead sperm.

Recipe: goat — testicle pill

kidney and testes of a male goat	one
Rhizoma Dioscoreae	80 g
Fructus Lycii	80 g
Herba Cistanchis	80 g
Radix Morindae Officinalis	80 g
Radix Rehmanniae Praeparata	80 g
Herba Epimedii	60 g
Semen Cuscutae	60 g
Fructus Corni	50 g
Fructus Schisandrae	30 g
Radix Angelicae Sinensis	40 g

Modification: For cases with emphasis on *yang* deficiency in the kidney, *Radix Aconiti Nigri* 30 g, *Cortex Cinnamomi* 50 g are added; for cases with emphasis on *yin* deficiency in the kidney, *Herba Epimedii* and *Semen Cuscutae* are omitted, and *Radix Rehmanniae* 80 g, *Rhizoma Anemarrhenae* 60 g, *Semen Plantaginis* 60 g, *Rhizoma Alismatis* 60 g, *Rhizoma Dioscoreae Septemlobae* 80 g are added; for blockage of *qi* associated with swelling pain in the testicles, *Radix Linderae* 60 g, *Fructus Foeniculi* 50 g, *Fructus Meliae Toosendan* 50 g, *Radix Bupleuri* 50 g, *Radix Paeoniae Alba* 70 g are added; for deficiency of *qi* or weak activity and low active rate of sperm, *Radix Astragali seu Hedysari* 120 g, *Radix Codonopsis Pilosulae* 100 g, *Fructus Psoraleae* 80 g are added.

Administration: The *kidney*, *ureter* and *testicle* of two — to four — year — old male goat is selected and soaked in salt water for 3 to 7 days (without washing). After the organs have been taken out of the salt water, they are dried in the sun, then cut into slices and baked further until the slices are completely dried. The dried slices are ground into powder which is mixed with honey and the powder of all above drugs to make pills (at 9 g each). 2 – 4 pills are taken daily with light salt water. The completion of all pills made from one dose of the above formula formed a course of treatment.

24 cases were treated with the above pills. After 1 – 4 courses of treatment, 16 cases were cured; 6 cases showed considerable improvement.

3. Infertility caused by recessive inflammation

Recipe:

Herba Taraxaci	10 g
Herba Hedyotis Diffusae	10 g
Caulis Sargentodoxae	10 g
Herba Violae	10 g
Rhizoma Achyranthis Bidentatae	10 g
Semen Vaccariae	10 g
Poria	10 g
Rhizoma Alismatis	10 g
Semen Plantaginis (decocted after being wrapped in a piece of cloth)	10 g
Caulis Bambusae in Taeniam	10 g
Semen Cuscutae	10 g
Radix Dipsaci	10 g
Fructus Lycii	10 g
Radix Polygoni Multiflori	10 g
Radix Salviae Miltiorrhizae	15 g
Radix Glycyrrhizae	4 g

Modification: *Herba Epimedii* is added for hyposexuality; *Herba Ecliptae*, *Fructus Ligustri Lucidi* are added for excessive red cells in the prostate or seminal fluid.

166 cases were treated with the above prescription. These cases include 98 cases with chronic prostatitis, 40 cases with chronic vesiculitis, 11 cases with epididymitis, 2 cases with epididymis tuberculosis, 3 cases with chronic inflamma-

tion of spermatogenic tubule and 19 cases with chronic reproductive infection of T
— mycoplasma. All of them were of abnormal sperm. As a result, 64 cases were
cured completely; 55 cases revealed considerable improvement. The total effective rate was 94.6%.

Other Therapies

Acupuncture and Moxibustion

1) non — ejaculation
Points: Qūgǔ(RN2), Zúwǔlǐ(LR10), Sānyīnjiāo(SP6).
Manipulation: The patient is requested to urinate and void the bladder before treatment. A filiform needle of 3 cun is inserted at point Zúwǔlǐ(LR10) and a filiform needle of 2 cun is inserted at point Qūgǔ(RN2). The sensation at Zúwǔlǐ (LR10) is required to reach the perineum; the needle is twisted in Qūgǔ(RN2) until the patient feels a sensation of soreness, numbness and distention in his lower abdomen and vulva; the needling sensation of Sānyīnjiāo(SP6) is required to make the patient feel soreness, numbness and distention in the medial of the leg. If the penis erected for a long period of time, Tàichōng(LR3) is added to clear the smoldering fire in the liver meridian; if impotence occurred, Tàixī(KI3), Zhàohǎi (KI6), Cìliáo(BL32) are pierced and moxibustion is applied to Shénquè(RN8), Guānyuán(RN4) in the mean time. Needles remain in all the points for 30 minutes. Treatment is given once a day. One course of treatment consists of 10 days. There is an interval of one week between two consecutive courses.

130 cases were treated with the above method. 118 cases were cured, and the curative rate was 90.7%; 93 cases of them were cured within one course of treatment, accounting for 78.9% of all the cured cases.

2) non — ejaculation
Point: Yǒngquán(KI1).
Manipulation: The patient is instructed to lie in a supine position with his legs straightened. The skin of point Yǒngquán(KI1) is sterilized routinely and punctured rapidly with a filiform of 1.5 cun at a perpendicular depth of 1 cun. Manipulation of strong stimulation is applied for the purpose of attenuation. It is appropriate to have the needling sensation radiate to the external genitals. After being twisted for 2 — 3 minutes, the needle is retained in the point for a total of

30 minutes. During the insertion time, the needle is twisted every 10 minutes. After the withdrawal of the needle, the doctor instructed patient to lie in a supine position without moving and to relax his whole body and adjust his breathing evenly. Putting one palm on the other hand, the doctor then massages the patient from the xiphoid to the symphysis, and from the medial of the thigh to the genital organ for 10 times. Afterwards, the patient is ordered to stand up with his feet at shoulder width; the doctor uses his fist to pound gently and deeply the patient's waist and the bilateral regions of the kidney 30 times respectively with dorsal palm. The treatment is given once a day. 7 times of treatment consisted of one course of therapy.

42 cases were treated with the above method. 35 cases were cured (presence of orgasm and capacity of smooth ejaculation), accounting for 83.3%.

2. *Nidus Vespae* 10 g and *Radix Angelicae Dahuricae* 10 g are baked dry to a crisp, then ground into fine powder which is mixed with vinegar to form a dough. The dough is smoothed on the navel upon which a piece of gauze is placed and fixed with adhesive tape. This treatment is given once a day or once every other day for a continuation of 3 – 5 times. Most of the patients will be cured after 5 – 7 times of the treatment.

Chapter Twenty
Carcinoma of Kidney, Renal Pelvis and Ureter

ETIOLOGY AND PATHOGENESIS

Of all malignant tumors, 1 – 2% cases belong to carcinoma of kidney, renal pelvis and ureter. Over 70% of patients are between 40 to 60 years old. The proportion of men to women is three to one. Although the location of each of the three carcinomas is different, their symptoms, diagnosis and treatment are basically the same, with only minor differences. They are therefore to be discussed as a group. The cause of these neoplasms is not clear. it has been speculated that chronic stimulation of kidney stones might induce carcinoma of renal pelvis and ureter. When irritating carcinogenous substances such as cigarettes or antipyretic analgesic phenacetin are used for a prolonged period, the incidence of carcinoma is high. With the weakening of kidney *qi* and *yin* – *yang* balance, due to advanced age the defense against internal and external carcinogenic factors, an important intrinsic factor of the patient, is not effective.

Macroscopic morphology usually displays an irregular lobulated tumor. The majority of carcinoma of the renal pelvis present a papillary structure, a minor group of which are solid induration. Under microscope, kidney carcinomas are divided into: hyaluronic cell carcinoma, granulocytic carcinoma, papillocarcinoma and undifferentiated carcinoma. Carcinoma of renal pelvis and ureter of the upper pole of right kidney are mostly solid papilloma. Most kidney carcinoma involve unilateral kidney, particularly the lateral upper pole of right kidney. Neoplasm spreads along the lymph node system around the aorta in most cases, then continues to spread to lungs, liver, bone and brain. Kidney carcinoma rarely extends to the ureter and urinary bladder, while renal pelvis carcinoma frequently spreads along the ureter and urinary bladder. It is considered possible that papillocarcinoma of renal pelvis, urinary bladder and ureter occur in response to the same carcinogenous substance, as the onset of these diseases are not due to metastasis.

MAIN SYMPTOMS AND SIGNS

The typical symptoms of this neoplasm are painless hematuria, lumbar or epigastric tumor mass and lumbago.

Hematuria: Bleeding after rupture of neoplasm's surface. The microscopic hematuria will cease after consecutive paroxysm for several days. The microscopic hematuria follows, and sometimes disappears. The hematuria occurs intermittently, and the interval between two paroxysms varies by several days, several weeks or several months. Although painless hematuria is characteristic of this neoplasm. When the bleeding is severe and occurs with carcinoma of renal pelvis, a blood clot or a long cord of thrombus is formed in the ureter, causing disturbance in urination. At times kidney and ureter colic occur.

Lumbo-Abdominal Tumor Mass: This is the symptom of the advanced stage. When the tumor is large, particularly when located at the lower pole, it is easy to detect. If the tumor mass is solid, it moves up and down in compliance with respiration. If it is fixed, it indicates there is infiltration and adhesion with adjacent tissues.

Lumbago: This symptom appears after hematuria and the tumor mass. A rare cause is traction of the tumor mass to the renal capsule or the involvement of perirenal tissue, which causes a dull pain in the region of the kidney, back and epigastrium.

The above three typical symptoms do not appear simultaneously, and the rate of appearance varies according to the difference in condition, course and location of lesions of the disease. Hematuria occurs in 57% of renal carcinoma, and with 90% of renal pelvis carcinomas; 54% of renal and renal pelvis carcinomas have lumbo-abdominal tumor masses and around 30% have lumbago.

When there is metastasis, corresponding symptoms are evoked. When it spreads to the brain, headache and symptoms of cranial hypertension appear; metastasis to the bone and spine induces pain in limbs and lumbocrural pain. The stimulation of oncogenic toxin and infection of tumor tissue, fever, emaciation, anemia, insomnia, a restlessness, thirst, constipation, dark urine, anorexia and symptoms of systemic exhaustion.

MAIN POINTS OF DIAGNOSIS

1. Symptoms

If the three typical symptoms, namely, hematuria, lumbo-abdominal tumor mass, and lumbago appear simultaneously, the disease in the advanced stage and there is no difficulty in establishing a diagnosis. If the above symptoms appear singly, one should be alert, and a comprehensive investigation is necessary.

2. X-ray film

1) **Abdominal X-ray**: A successful supine positioned abdominal picture displays the enlargement of kidney shadow, with an irregular and prominent margin; change of kidney location, deviation of the angle between longitudinal axis of kidney and reno-spinal angle. Due to increase in size of tumor, neoplasm located at the upper pole of kidney, have two longitudinal axles which tend to be parallel, and the reno-spinal angel is less than 15 degrees. With tumor of lower pole, the reno-spinal angel is greater than 25°, because the kidney is being pushed outward by the tumor.

2) **Intravenous Urography**: Shows picture of kidney, its contour and margin, and it can be observed, it the renal calyces are compressed, dilated or constricted.

3) **Abdominal Aortography**: Abdominal aortography and perirenal inflation radiography are helpful to a certain extent.

4) **Injecting Contrast Medium Intravenously**: Nephrotomography is helpful differentiating between neoplasm and cyst. This method has now been replaced by **B ultrasonography**.

3. cystoscopic examination and retrograde radiography

These methods are used to observe the ejection of blood from orifice of ureter to clarify the source of hematuria. With retrograde radiography, the filling condition of renal pelvis, calyces and ureter is monitored and is important in establishing a diagnosis.

4. B ultrasonography

The sonograms of renal carcinoma and benign tumor, cyst and hydronephrosis are simple to differentiate. Ultrasonography possesses the advantage of being painless, non-invasive, inexpensive and relatively accurate when compared with intravenous urography, retrograde radiography and **CT scanning**. It may not be accurate when diagnosing neoplasm of renal pelvis and ureter, **X-ray** film, intravenous and retrograde radiography are therefore still necessary for establishing a diagnosis.

5. CT scanning

This method can show size of tumor, extent of infiltration to adjacent organs, and supplements the inadequacy of other investigations, but is difficult to use for a qualitative assessment.

6. laboratory findings

1) Microscopic Examination of Urine: Microscopic hematuria usually occur before or after microscopic hematuria, and may persist for a long period, or disappear spontaneously with or without treatment. Three Glass Test is implemented to assess which section of urinary tract the urinary erythrocytes come from.

2) Cancer Cells in Urine: Positivity is high when technical conditions are good, otherwise false negativity is also high.

7. radioactive isotope scanning

Scanning is capable of discriminating shape, size and location of neoplasm, but has already been replaced by **B ultrasonography**.

DIFFERENTIATION AND TREATMENT OF COMMON SYNDROMES

Therapeutic measures of traditional Chinese medicine and Western medicine should be selected to implement combined therapy, according to indications of different conditions, stage, severity and exigency of the disease. Treatment by traditional Chinese medicine should be implemented throughout entire therapeutic course, regardless of what it is based on. This not only creates favorable conditions for chemotherapy, but reduces sides side effects as well, and displays the crucial role of eliminating and inhibiting residual tumor.

1. hematuria due to damp-heat accumulation in kidney

Most patients are "first visitors" to the doctor and have not received any aggressive treatment or have been treated with conservative therapy, with no apparent effect.

Main Symptoms and Signs: Painless hematuria appear intermittently, protracts for several months with no further effects, or lumbodorsal aching pain, lump in abdomen or lumbar region, with low fever at times, fatigue and lassitude, mild anorexia, red tongue with white greasy coating yellow in center, rapid, slippery or thready pulse.

Therapeutic Principles: Clear up the dampness and heat, detoxicate and resolve the stasis.

Recipe:

Herba Solanii Lyrati	20 g
Herba Duchesneae Indicae	20 g
Herba Solani Nigri	20 g
Rhizoma Imperatae	15 g
Herba Agrimoniae	18 g
Polyporus	15 g
Poria	12 g
Talcum	15 g
Herba Polygoni Avicularis	18 g
Semen Coicis	18 g
Radix Glycyrrhizae	6 g
Rhizoma Atractylodis Macrocephalae	10 g

2. Residual toxin remains uncleared after treatment

Corresponding to side effects, sequelae after surgery, chemotherapy or radiotherapy. Residual tumor still remaining in body.

Main Symptoms and Signs: After surgery, chemotherapy or radiotherapy, tumor is inhibited, but qi is impaired, and manifests soreness of the waist and weakness in legs, listlessness, occasional low fever or hematuria, leukopenia, and often anemia, or anorexia, pale red or pale white tongue with thin white greasy coating, soft and powerless or thready and rapid pulse.

Therapeutic Principles: Nourish the kidney and invigorate the spleen, strengthen the body resistance and remove pathogenic factors.

Recipe:

Radix Codonopsis	15 g
Rhizoma Atractylodis Macrocephalae	12 g
Poria	12 g
Radix Glycyrrhizae	3 g
Fructus Lycii	10 g
Radix Pseudostellariae	15 g
Radix Rehmanniae Praeparata	15 g
Radix Astragali seu Hedysari	15 g
Radix Ophiopogonis	12 g
Herba Agrimoniae	18 g
Herba Scutellariae Barbatae	
Radix Cirsii Japonici and Herba Cirsii	30 g
Polyporus	12 g
Spora Lygodii	10 g
Herba Dianthi	10 g

3. **stagnancy of** *blood* **and** *yin* **deficiency of liver and kidney**

In middle or advanced stage or after chemotherapy, radiotherapy or surgery, manifests heat reaction or relapse.

Main Symptoms and Signs: Frequent episodes of hematuria, dull pain around waist, lump in abdomen or lumbar region enlarging day by day, or recurrence of tumor after surgical excision, resulting in dry mouth and tongue, constipation, restlessness and insomnia, heat sensation on palms, and soles due to impairment of *yin*, the result of protracted disease, chemotherapy or radiotherapy. Tongue is red with some coating, or crimson red, or red purple, smooth and uncoated or with coating, thready, rapid or taut pulse.

Therapeutic Principles: Nourish *yin* and replenish the kidney, dissolve the stasis and lump.

Recipe:

Radix Ophiopogonis	12 g
Radix Asparagi	15 g
Radix Glehniae	12 g
Herba Dendrobii	12 g

Rhizoma Anemarrhenae	10 g
Fructus Lycii	12 g
Radix Pseudostellariae	15 g
Rhizoma Polygonati	12 g
Fructus Ligustri Lucidi	15 g
Radix Cirsii Japonici and *Herba Cirsii*	30 g
Herba Agrimoniae	20 g
Herba Solanii Lyrati	20 g
Polyporus	15 g
Rhizoma Atractylodis Macrocephalae	10 g
Radix Paeoniae Rubra	10 g
Rhizoma Gynostemmatis Pentaphylli	15 g
Radix Panacis Quinquefolii	6 g

4. **spreading of cancer and deficiency of** *qi* **and** *blood*

Advanced stage with remote metastasis, with no ameliorating effects from various treatments, or with relapse after remission, or patient already in advanced stage on first visit.

Main Symptoms and Signs: Fatigue and weakness, spontaneous sweating and night sweat sallow complexion, occasional hematuria, lumbago, flatulence, anemia, emaciation, shortness of breath on exertion, at times a cough, accompanied by low fever, dry mouth, no desire for drink, pale red or dark purple tongue with petechia, thready weak or feeble, wide and rapid pulse.

Therapeutic Principles: Nourish both *qi* and *blood*, strengthen the body resistance and inhibit the tumor.

Recipe:

Radix Astragali seu Hedysari	25 g
Radix Pseudostellariae	18 g
Radix Codonopsis	12 g
Poria	12 g
Rhizoma Atractylodis Macrocephalae	12 g
Radix Glycyrrhizae	3 g
Radix Ophiopogonis	12 g
Radix Asparagi	12 g
Radix Rehmanniae	15 g

Radix Rehmanniae Praeparata	15 g
Fructus Lycii	10 g
Fructus Ligustri Lucidi	12 g
Rhizoma Polygonati	12 g
Flos Lonicerae	9 g
Herba Agrimoniae	18 g
Radix Panacis Quinquefolii Lateralis	6 g

prescription for carcinoma with hematuria complicated by infection

Recipe:

Semen Coicis	30 g
Spora Lygodii	15 g
Herba Scutellariae Barbatae	30 g
Herba Lobetiae Chinensis	20 g
Rhizoma Imperatae	15 g
Herba Chenopodii Hybridi	
Radix Cirsii Japonici&Herba Cirsii	20 g
Poria	15 g
Rhizoma Atractylodis Macrocephalae	12 g
Rhizoma Dioscoreae	10 g
Radix Codonopsis	10 g
Radix Glycyrrhizae	3 g
Radix Scutellariae	
Herba Dianthi	15 g

All the above drugs are to be decocted in water for oral administration.

Combining TCM with Surgery

Surgery is the major measure for treatment of cancer, a radical cure for early cases and a palliative treatment in intermediate and advanced stages. When planning an effective program for surgery, the following should be taken into account: stage of illness, severity of illness, differences in biological characteristics of tumor cells, general condition of patient, degree of deviation of *yin* - *yang* balance, the appropriate integrated medical treatment, as well as the skill and experience of the surgeon.

1. pre-operative integrated traditional Chinese medicine therapy

It is generally recognized that cancer is a local manifestation of a general ailment. Once a tumor mass exists, there will be manifestations of *yin-yang* disharmony. By applying TCM diagnostic measures, syndromes can be differentiated and treatment given in time, keeping the patient in general good health, ready for surgery. First the patient is given the subsequent recipe to nourish the *yin* and reduce the adverse ascending *qi* to stop nausea.

Recipe:

 fRadix Astragali seu Hedysari
 Radix Codonopsis
 Rhizoma Atractylodis Macrocephalae
 Poria
 Radix Glycyrrhizae
 Fructus Evodiae
 Rhizoma Coptidis
 Radix Ophiopogonis
 Radix Glehniae
 Radix Pseudostellariae
 Rhizoma Anemarrhenae
 Herba Dendrobii
 Fructus Trichosanthis
 Calyx Kaki
 Pericarpium Citri Reticulatae
 Flos Inulae
 Haematitum

A few days later, the patient may take the following prescription.

Recipe: *Jianpi liqi tang*

Radix Codonopsis	10 g
Rhizoma Atractylodis Macrocephalae	9 g
Poria	12 g
Radix Astragali seu Hedysari	12 g
Radix Ophiopogonis	10 g
Radix Aucklandiae	6 g
Radix Glehniae	10 g
Pericarpium Citri Reticulatae	6 g

Semen Trichosanthis	15 g
Semen Nelumbinis	15 g
Endothelium Corneum Gigeriae Galli	9 g
Fructus Hordei et Setariae Germinatus	30 g
Massa Medicata Fermentata	9 g
Rhizoma Coptidis	4.5 g
Radix Glycyrrhizae	3 g

All the above drugs are to be decocted in water for oral administration.

2. integrated traditional Chinese medicine treatment after surgery

Grave consequences and heavy burdens can develop for the patient as the result of surgical wounds, defective organs, loss of blood and fluid, anesthesia, pain insomnia, and loss of appetite. Different syndromes appear according to the degree of organic damage and the choice of surgery. This may include disturbance of gastrointestinal functions, disharmony of ying and wei, defective superficial defense mechanism, disappearance of body fluids, thirst, or constipation and should be treated accordingly.

1) regulation of the function of spleen and stomach

Apply *Jianpi liqi tang*, one dose beginning the 4th day after surgery, and continuing with 3 to 7 successive doses. The remedy should be taken frequently, as it also alleviates side effects, and other complications and shortens the time needed for hospitalization.

2) traditional Chinese medicine and consolidating the superficies

After surgery some patients reveal profuse asthenic sweating whenever they move, are chilly after sweating and experience general malaise. This is due to disharmony of ying and wei, which leaves a state of asthenic superficies and should be treated with *yupingfeng san* to consolidate the superficies. The modified recipe is as follows:

Recipe:

Radix Astragali seu Hedysari
Radix Saposhinkoviae
Rhizoma Atractylodis Macrocephalae
Fructus Schisandrae
Fructus Tritici Levis
Concha Ostreae

Radix Codonopsis
Radix Paeoniae Alba
Radix Glycyrrhizae

All the above drugs are to be decocted in water for oral administration.

3) **nourishing yin to produce body fluid**

When no post-operative complications occur, thirsts and a dry mouth with fever will subside spontaneously after one week. If these symptoms persist longer and include constipation, uncoated crimson tongue, restlessness, coughing, shortness of breath and fever, it usually indicates infection, such as bronchial pneumonia, pyothorax, anastomose fistula, hydrothorax, local purulent abdomen, subphrenic abscess, foreign body in the cavity, urinary or biliary infections, bacteremia or septicemia. This is due to *yin*-damage caused by the surgical wound, and should be treated with massive doses of herbs capable of nourishing the *yin*.

Recipe:

Radix Panacis Quinquefolii
Radix Pseudostellariae
Radix Panacis Quinquefolii Lateralis
Radix Ginseng
Herba Dendrobii
Rhizoma Polygonati Odorati
Rhizoma Anemarrhenae
Poria
Polyporus
Radix Scutellariae
Radix Rehmanniae
Nodus Nelumbinis Rhizomatis
Rhizoma Imperatae
Rhizoma Polygonati
Radix Paeoniae Alba
Cortex Moutan
Fructus Trichosanthis
Tremmella

All the above drugs are to be decocted in water for oral administration.

Chapter Twenty-one
Commonly Used Recipes

Anti-inflammatory and Analgesic Bolus
(Pian Zi Huang)

Ingredients

Not yet pubished. 0.3 g each piece, or slice, 0.6 g each packet.

Administration and Dosage

To be taken orally, children: 1-8 years, 0.15-0.3 g; over 8 years and adults, 0.6 g each time. Twice or three times a day. External Use, for original appearance of black or white vesiculae of innominate inflammatory swelling, mix one or two slices of *Pian Zi Huang* with cold boiled water or vinegar and apply it to the affected area; in case of ulceration, apply it to the perripheral area several times a day to keep local dampness.

Efficacy

Clearing away heat and toxic materials, relicving swelling and pain.

Indications

Acute or chronic hepatitis, tympanitis, gum abscess, oral ulcer, bee sting, snakebite, nail-like boil and innominate inflammatory swelling.

Anti-inflammatory Pill
(Liu Ying Wan)

Ingredients

Margarita
Calculus Bovis
Venenum Bufonis
Pills, 100 pills per bottle.

Efficacy

Clearing away heat and toxic material, subduing swelling and pain.

Indications

Tonsillitis, furuncle, sore, diseases of throat, the bite of insects, etc..

Administration and Dosage

To be taken orally with boiled water. Adults: 10 pills each time; children: 5 pills each time; infants: 2 pills each time, 3 times a day.

For external use, disintegrate some pills in just a little cold boiled water or vinegar and then apply it to the affected part of skin.

Cautions

Never to be administered to pregnant women.

Acanthopanax Infusion
(Wujiashen Chongji)

INGREDIENTS

Radix Acanthopanacis Senticosi

Process

Make medicinal cubes (infusion), 25 g each cube.

Actions

Strengthening the body resistance and restoring normal functions of the body to consolidate the constitution, relieving mental stress and promoting intelligence.

INDICATIONS

Insomnia, excessive dreadming, fatigue and weakness, poor appetite and others caused by neurosis and other diseases. It has certain effects in relieving angina pectoris of coronary heart disease. It is also used for the treatment of leukopenia.

Direction

To be taken orally after being infused in boiling water, one cube eahc time, twice daily.

Banlong Pill
(Ban Long Wan)

INGREDIENTS

Colla Cornu Cervi	10 g
Poria	10 g
Semen Biotae	10 g
Semen Cuscutae	10 g
Fructus Psoraleae	10 g
Pulvis Cornu Cervi	20 g
Radix Rehmanniae Praeparata	20 g

EFFICACY

Nourishing and invigorating the kidney - essence, preserving sperm and tranquilizing; mainly for cases of nocturnal emission, impotence or premature ejaculation accompanied with lumbago, tinnitus, nocturia, dizziness, fatigue, pale complexion, pale tongue with white fur, sunken and small, weak pulse, which are attributive to the impairment of kidney - essence and weakness of kidney qi.

INDICATIONS

1. Applicable to cases of prolonged metrorrhagia or leucorrhagia, accompanied with dizziness, lumbago, weakness of the knee joints, spiritlessness, pale tongue with whitish fur, feeble pulse, which are attributive to insufficiency of essential substance and blood and weakness of kidney qi.

2. For cases with spontaneous flow of thin breast milk after delivery, shortness of breath, fatigue, lumbago, dimmish complexion, pale tongue with whitish fur, sunken and feeble pulse, which are attributive to insufficiency of kidney - essence and deficiency of kidney qi.

3. Also applicable to cases of hypothyroidism, neurasthenia, Addison's disease, dysfunctional uterine bleeding, hysteromyoma and endometritis, which are attributive to insufficiency of essential substance and blood, and deficiency of kid-

ney qi.

INTERPRETATION

Colla Cornu Cervi not only invigorates essential substance and blood but also warms and strengthens kidney yang, and serves as the principal drug of the prescription. Radix Rehmanniae Praeparata and Semen Cuscutae can benefit yin and invigorate yang, which tonifies the essential substances, blood and kidney – yang when it is used together with Colla Cornu Cervi. Fructus Psoraleae acts with Colla Cornu Cervi to invigorate kidney and strengthen yang. Semen Biotae used together with Poria serves to keep heart – fire and kidney – water in balance, and tranquilize the patient. Fructus Psoraleae enhances the emission – relieving effect of Cornu Cervi.

Baolong Pill
(Baolong Wan)

INGREDIENTS

Concretio Silicae Bambusae	30 g
Realgar	3 g
Cinnabaris	15 g
Moschus	15 g
Rhizoma Arisaema cum Bile	

120 g PROCESS: *Grind the above ingredients into powder to make pills.*

EFFICACY

Clearing away heat, dispersing phlegm, relieving convulsion and fainting; mainly for infants with convulsive seizures attributive to accumulation of phlegm – heat, which manifest as fever, somnolence or loss of consciousness, rough breathing, convulsion, red tongue with yellow, turbid and greasy fur.

INDICATIONS

1. Because the prescription contains Realgar and Moschus, it should not be boiled and prepared as decoction.
2. Applicable to infants with convulsion resulting from high fever, accompanied with red tongue and yellow fur, wiry and smooth pulse.
3. Also indicated for cases with epileptic seizures accompanied with yellow, turbid and greasy fur on the tongue, which are attributive to blockage of the orifices by phlegm - heat.
4. Also applicable to cases of uremic coma, hepatic coma and hysteria attributive to accumulation of phlegm - heat; and to cases of encephalitis B, epidemic meningitis, thermoplegia and cerebral malaria marked by high fever and convulsion, which are attributive to attack of severe heat and wind.

INTERPRETATION

Concretio Silicae Bambusae has the effects of clearing away heat, eliminating phlegm, cooling heart - fire and relieving convulsion. Arisaema cum Bile can disperse phlegm, suppress wind and relieve convulsion. The combination of two serves as the principal drugs for the treatment of convulsion of phlegm - heat type. Realgar can eliminate phlegm and toxic material. Moschus is used for waking up the patient from unconsciousness, and Cinnabaris for tranquilizing. The last three drugs together exert a strong anti - convulsive and resuscitating effect.

Bolus for Activating Meridians
(Huo Luo Dan)

INGREDIENTS

Radix Aconiti Praeparata	6 g
Radix Aconiti Kusnezoffii Praeparata	6 g
Lumbricus	10 g

Rhizoma Arisaema cum Bile Praeparata	10 g
Olibanum	3 g
Myrrha	3 g

EFFICACY

Warming the channels, activating the circulation of collaterals, expelling wind evil, eliminating dampness and phlegm and removing blood stasis; mainly for cases with prolonged numbness and pain of the extremities, atttributive to retention of wind-phlegm and blood stasis in the meridians.

INDICATIONS

1. Applicable to cases of arthralgia of wind - cold - dampness type manifested as prolonged immobility and pain of joints, numbness of muscles and skin, white and greasy fur on the tongue, wiry and smooth pulse.

2. Also applicable to cases of stroke attributive to obstruction of meridians by wind-phlegm, which are manifested as hemiplegia, spasm of limbs, white and greasy fur on the tongue and wiry pulse.

3. Also applicable to cases of Guillain - Barre syndromes, plexus brachialis neuralgia, ischialgia, multiple neuritis, etc., marked by pain of limbs, which are attributive to obstruction of meridians by wind-phlegm and blood stasis, or cases of reheumatic arthritis and cerebral accidents, which are attributive to attack of wind-cold-dampness or obstruction of the meridians by wind-phlegm.

INTERPRETATION

Radix Aconiti Praeparata and Radix Aconiti Kusnezoffii Praeparata can warm the channels, activate the circulation of collaterals and elimintae cold dampness evil from the meridians, and also expel wind evil and relieve pain. Rhizoma Arisaema cum Bile Praeparata can expel wind-phlegm from the meridians, relieve spasm and pain. The above three drugs constituent an effective remedy for eliminating wind-phlegm and blood stasis from meridians. Olibanum and Myrrha serve to disperse blood stasis from the meridians, and the wine can enhance their effects. Lumbricus is helpful to dredge and activate the meridians. In sum, the prescription aims at eliminating wind-phlegm and blood stasis from the meridians, and then relieving pain.

Bolus for Severe Endogenous Wind-Syndrome
(Da Ding Feng Zhu)

INGREDIENTS

Radix Paeoniae Alba	18 g
Radix Rehmanniae	18 g
Colla Corii Asini	10 g
Radix Ophiopogonis	10 g
Plastrum Testudinis	12 g
Concha Ostreae	12 g
Carapax Trionycis	12 g
Semen Sesami	6 g
Fructus Schisandrae	6 g
Radix Glycyrrhizae Praeparata	3 g
Fresh egg yolk	1

EFFICACY

Nourishing yin and calming wind, mainly for cases of clonic convulsion attributive to damge of true-yin by heat and hyperactivity of liver-wind, which are accompanied with listlessness, crimson and uncoated tongue, small and weak pulse.

INDICATIONS

1. Indicated for cases attributive to deficiency of liver-yin and kidney-yin and upward attack of liver-yang, which are manifested as dizziness aggravated

by over strain or anger, soreness of the loin and knees, insomnia and dreaminess, nocturnal emission, fatigue, bright red tongue, small and rapid pulse.

2. Also applicable to cases of encephalitis B, epidemic meningitis, poliomyelitis and chorea, marked by convulsion, which are attributive to damage of true-yin by heat and hyperactivity of liver-wind.

INTERPRETATION

Egg yolk and Colla Corii Asini are applied to nourish yin-fluid, supplement the exhausted true-yin and calm liver-wind. Rehmanniae, Sesami, Ophiopogonis and Paeoniae Alba serve to nourish yin and blood, soothe the liver and calm wind. Plastrum Testudinis, Concha Ostreae and Carapax Trionycis can invigorate kidney-yin and suppress hyperactive liver-yang.

Radix Glycyrrhizae Praeparata and Fructus Schisandrae are helpful for yin nourishing and wind calming.

Bolus of Arisaematis
(Tiannanxing Wan)

INGREDIENTS

Arisaema cum Bile	10 g
Radix Angelicae Dahuriacae	10 g
Radix Ledebouriellae	10 g
Rhizoma et Radix Notopterygii	10 g
Radix Angelicae Pubescentis	10 g
Rhizoma Ligustici Chuanxiong	10 g
Rhizoma Gastrodiae 10 g	
Radix Paeoniae Alba	10 g
Bombyx Batryticatus	10 g
Herba Ephedrae	6 g
Radix Platycodi	6 g
Herba Asari	6 g

Radix Glycyrrhizae Praeparata	6 g
Rhizoma Zingiberis	6 g
Borneolum Syntheticum	3 g
Moschus	0.6 g

PROCESS: *All the above ingredients are to be prepared with honey as boluses.*

EFFICACY

Expelling wind evil and phlegm, waking up the patient and dredging the meridians; mainly for cases of stroke attributed to accumulation of wind-phlegm evil in the interior, which are manifested as numbness of limbs, hemiplegia, aphasia, whitish and greasy fur on the tongue, floating and smooth pulse.

INDICATIONS

1. Applicable to cases with swelling pain and immobility of joints, numbness of skin and muscle, whitish and greasy fur on the tongue, smooth pulse, which are attributed to artharalgia of wind-cold-dampness type.

2. Also applicable to cases of cerebral accidents, chronic rheumatic arthritis, sciatica, cervical vertebra syndrome, etc. manifested as hemiplegia, or arthralgia, or numbness of limbs, which are attributed to accumulation of wind-phlegm evil in the interior or arthralgia of wind-cold-dampness type.

INTERPRETATION

Arisaema cum Bile has a potent effect of expelling wind-phlegm evil and dredging the meridians, and acts as the chief drugs in the prescription. Bombyx Batryticatus enhances the effect of Arisaema cum Bile; Ledebouriellae, Notopterygii, Angelicae Pubescentis, Angelicae Dahuricae and Herba Menthae are helpful to expel wind evil and eliminate the dampness evil. Since phlegm-dampness evil is of yin nature, so Zingiberis and Asari are applied to warm the meridians and expel cold evil, and also help Arisaema cum Bile to dry the dampness and eliminate phlegm, so that the mobility of the extremities will be restored. Borneolum Syntheticum and Moschus have the effect of dredging the meridians, and are helpful to relieve aphasia. Gastrodiae, Glycyrrhizae Praeparata, Ligustici Chuanxiong and Paeoniae Alba have the effects of regulating vital energy and blood, subduing endogenous wind evil and relieving convulsion.

Bolus of Placenta Hominis
(Heche Ba Wei Wan)

INGREDIENTS

Placenta Hominis	1 set (cooked with ginger juice and wine)
Fructus Corni	30 g
Radix Ophiopogonis	30 g
Radix Rehmanniae Praeparata	90 g
(cooked with ginger juice and Fructus Amomi)	
Cortex Moutan Radicis	15 g
Rhizoma Alismatis	15 g
Cornu Cervi Pantotrichum	60 g
Fructus Schisandrae	60 g
Rhizoma Dioscoreae	165 g
Poria	45 g
Radix Aconiti Praeparata	22 g
Ramulus Cinnamomi	22 g

PROCESS: *Grind the above ingredients into powder to make pills with honey.*

EFFICACY

Invigorating kidney, benefiting essence and vital energy and nourishing blood; mainly for cases attributive to impairment of kidney - energy and insufficiency of lung and spleen qi after epileptic seizures, which manifest as spiritlessness, dizziness, palpitation, lumbago, fatigue of the lower limbs, aversion to cold, weakness, poor appetite, loose stools, pale and corpulent tongue with white and smooth fur, slow and weak pulse.

INDICATIONS

1. Indicated for infantile maldevelopment manifested by tardiness of ability to walk, delayed growth of the teeth, weakness of the tendon and bone, pale tongue with white fur, sunken and weak pulse, which are attributive to insufficiency of kidney-yang.

2. Also for cases of sterility, impotence or nocturnal emission accompanied with dizziness, tinnitus, lumbago, cold limbs, pale and corpulent tongue with white and smooth fur, which are attributive to the impairment of kidney-yang and insufficiency of essence and blood.

3. Applicable to cases of leukorrhagia with profuse thin discharge, lumbago, fatigue, feeling of coldness over the lower abdomen, nocturia, spiritlessness, which are attributive to the weakness of kidney qi and loss of essence fluid.

4. Also applicable to cases of senile dementia and climacterium syndrome with spiritlessness, which are attributive to the impairment of kidney qi and insufficiency of lung and spleen qi; and to cases of endometritis and senile vaginitis with leukorrhagia, which are attributive to weakness of kidney qi and loss of essence substance.

INTERPRETATION

The prescription is formed by adding Placenta Hominis, Ophiopogonis, Cornu Cervi Pantotrichum and Schisandrae to Pill for Invigorating Kidney Qi which has the effects of invigorating kidney yin, nourishing liver blood, benefiting spleen yin and strengthening kidney yang. Ophiopogonis and Schisandrae used together with the Boluses serves to nourish the lung and kidney. Cornu Cervi Pantotrichum is used for promoting the production of essence and marrow and benefiting qi. Placenta Hominis has a strong effect of tonifying qi and blood, and is available for various kinds of conscumptive diseases.

Bolus of Precious Drugs
(Zhi Bao Dan)

INGREDIENTS

Cornu Rhinocerotis	30 g
Carapax Eretmochelydis	30 g
Succinum	30 g
Cinnabaris	30 g
Realgar	30 g
Borneolum Syntheticum	0.3 g
Moschus	0.3 g
Calculus Bovis	15 g
Benzoinum	45 g
Gold sheet	50 pcs (half for coating)
Silver sheet	50 pcs

PROCESS: *All the above drugs are ground into powder and prepared into boluses, each weighs 3 g.*

EFFICACY

Eliminating dampness - phlegm, waking up patients from unconsciousness, clearing away heart - fire and detoxifying; mainly for cases of coma, profuse expectoration, heavy breath, fever, restlessness, red tongue with yellowish, greasy and dirty fur, smooth and rapid pulse, which are attributive to the attack of the interior by heat evil and stagnation of dampness - phlegm, also for the infantile convulsion due to stagnation of phlegm - heat.

INDICATIONS

1. Applicable to cases of sudden fainting or apoplexy attributive to the attack of percardium by phlegm - heat although there is no fever.

2. Applicable to cases of sunstroke attributive to stagnation of dampness - phlegm and retention of summer - heat.

3. It has been recorded in Prescription of People's Welfare Pharmacy that

the bolus is taken with ginger juice to enhance the effect of waking up a patient.

4. Also applicable to comatose cases of hepatic coma, cerebrovascular accident, epilepsy, uremia, etc. which are attributive to retention of heat and dampness – phlegm.

INTERPRETATION

Calculus Bovis can eliminate phlegm, wake up one from unconciousness, clear away heart – fire and has the effect of detoxication. Its action is strong and rapid, so it is used as the principal drug. Moschu, Borneolum Syntheticum and Benzoinum have the effects of exorcising evils, dissipating dampness – phlegm and restoring consciousness; Cornu Rhinocerotis and Carapax Eretmochelydis can clear away heart – fire and have the action of detoxication. Realgar has the effect of detoxication and Cinnabaris, Succinum, gold sheet and silver sheet have the effect of tranquilizing. The combination of these drugs constitutes a prescription with eliminating dampness – phlegm and waking up one from unconsciousness as the chief effect, and with clearing away heart – fire and detoxifying as the auxiliary one. This is different from Bolus of Calculus Bovis for Resurrection.

Bolus of Storax
(Suhexiang Wan)

INGREDIENTS

Rhizoma Atractylodis Macrocephalae	60 g
Radix Aucklandiae	60 g
Cornu Rhinocerotis	60 g
Rhizoma Cyperi	60 g
Cinnabaris	60 g
Fructus Chebulae	60 g
Lignum Santali	60 g
Benzoinum	60 g
Lignum Aquilariae Resinatum	60 g

Moschus	60 g
Flos Caryophylli	60 g
Fructus Pipers Longi	60 g
Borneolum Syntheticum	30 g
Oleum Storax	30 g
Olibanumm'	30 g

PROCESS : *All the above ingredients are prepared with honey to make boluses.*

EFFICACY

Warming and dredging the meridians to wake up patients from unconsciousness. sciousness, promoting the circulation of vital energy and eliminating the dampness evil; mainly for cases due to the obstruction of vital energy circulation by Relieve cold or phlegm - dampness evil and impairment of consciousness, which are manifested as sudden syncope, lockjaw, cyanosis and pallor, cold breath, whitish and smooth fur on the tongue, sunken, slow and strong pulse.

INDICATIONS

1. Applicable to cases of angina pectoris attributive to stagnation of cold evil and vital energy or attack of dampness evil.

2. May be used as an emergency treatment for cases due to phlegm obstruction of the heart, manifested as epileptic seizures, mental upset, staring eyes, paraphasia, whitish and greasy fur on the tongue, before other causative treatments are applied.

3. Indicated only for cold type asthenia - syndrome of coma.

4. Also applicable to comatose cases of cerebral accidents, uremia, hepatic coma, etc.; mental disorders occuring in psychosis, such as schizophrenia, symptomatic psychosis, etc.; chest pain occuring in angina pectoris and myocardial infarction; which are attributive to the obstruction of vital energy circulation by cold or phlegm - dampness evil.

INTERPRETATION

This prescription is a typical preescription for waking up patient from unconsciousness, which composed of many aromatic drugs such as Storax, Benzoinum, Moschus and Borneolum Syntheticum, Cornu Rhinocerotis has the effects of clearing away heart – fire and eliminating toxic material; Cinnabaris, that of tranquilizing. The above six drugs used together are effective for waking up the patient from unconsciousness and for tranquilizing. Santali, Caryophylli, Cyperi, Aquilariae Resinatum, Pipers Longi, Boswelliae Olibanum and Atractylodis Macrocephalae constitute another group of herbs for regulating the function of viscera and enhancing the dampness – dispersing and waking effect. Chebulae of warm and astringing nature is added to prevent the damage of healthy energy by the aromatic drugs.

Brain – Invigorating and Kidney – Tonifying Pill
(Jian Nao Bu Shen Wan)

INGREDIENTS

Semen Ziziphi Spinosae
Radix Polygalae
Os Draconis Fossilia Ossis Mastodi
Radix Cyathulae
Cortex Eucommiae
Cinnabaris
Radix Angelicae Sinensis
Rhizoma Dioscoreae
Radix Ginseng
Cornu Cervi Pantotrichum

EFFICACY

Invigorating the brain, replenishing qi, tonifying the kidney and strengthening the essence of life.

INDICATIONS

Applicable to cases of neurosis, amnesia, insomnia, dizziness, vertigo, tinnitus, palpitation, lassitude in loin and knees, emission due to kidney deficiency, etc..

Cardiotonic Pill
(Tianwang Buxin Dan)

INGREDIENTS

Radix Rehmanniae	120 g
Radix Scrophulariae	60 g
Radix Salviae Miltiorrhizae	60 g
Radix Angelicae Sinensis	60 g
Radix Ginseng	60 g
Poria	60 g
Semen Biotae	60 g
Semen Ziziphi Spinosae	60 g
Radix Polygalae	60 g
Radix Asparagi	60 g
Radix Ophiopogonis	60 g
Fructus Schisandrae	60 g
Radix Platycodi	60 g

DIRECTIONS

Take 9 grams three times daily. It can also be made into decoction, with the dosage modified proportionally according to the original recipe.

EFFICACY

Nourishing yin to remove heat and tonifying blood to tranquilize the mind.

INDICATIONS

1. Asthenic fire stirring up inside due to deficiency of yin and blood brought on by the hypofunction of heart and kidney marked by insomnia with vexation, palpitation, mental weariness, nocturnal emission, amnesia, dry stools, orolingual boil, reddened tongue with little fur, thready and rapid pulse.

2. Neurosism, paroxysmal tachycardia, hypertension, hyperthyroidism and others marked by the above-mentioned symptoms can be treated by the modified recipe.

3. Modern researches have proved that the recipe has a better effect of regulating the cerebral cortex. It can tranquilize the mind to induce sleep without causing listlessness and achieve the effects of enriching the blood and relieving the symptoms of coronary heart disease.

CAUTIONS

The recipe is composed of nourishing, greasy drugs which affect the stomach, so it is not fit to take for a long time.

Decoction for Activating Blood Circulation
(Tong Qiao Huo Xue Tang)

INGREDIENTS

Radix Paeoniae Rubra	10 g
Rhizoma Ligustici Chuanxiong	10 g
Semen Persicae	10 g

Bulbus Allii Fistulosi 10 g
Rhizoma Zingiberis Recens   10 g
Flos Carthami   6 g
Fructus Ziziphi Jujubae   6 pcs
Moschus   0.3 g
wine q·s·

EFFICACY

Activating blood circulation and opening the orificies; mainly for cases of headache and dizziness due to accumulation of blood stasis in the head.

INDICATIONS

1. Indicated for cases of alopecia, deafness and sinusitis, which are attributive to accumulation of blood stasis in the head.

2. For cases of sudden loss of vision which are attributive to accumulation of blood stasis in the eyes, omit wine and Ziziphi Jujubae and add Faeces Vespertilionis and Radix Salviae Miltiorrhizae to nourish blood and promote vision.

3. Also applicable to sequelae of cerebral concussion, cases of cerebral arteriosclerosis and cerebellar bleeding with headache and dizziness, and to cases of retinal hemorrhage and embolism of central retinal artery with sudden loss of vision which are attributive to the same mechanism.

INTERPRETATION

Persicae, Carthami, Paeoniae Rubra and Ligustici Chuanxiong have the effects of activating blood circulation and removing blood stasis. Allii Fistulosi and Zingiberis help the above drugs distributing to the vertex. Moschus, fragrant and active, can dredge the passage of meridians and open the orifice, and is particularly suitable for the treatment of headache and dizziness due to accumulation of blood stasis in the head when used together with Persicae and Carthami. Wine and Ziziphi Jujubae used together have the effects of promoting blood flow and distributing the above drugs to the head.

Decoction for Eliminating Dampness and Relieving Rheumatism
(Chu Shi Juan Bi Tang)

INGREDIENTS

Rhizoma Atractylodis	12 g
Rhizoma Atractylodis Macrocephalae	10 g
Poria	10 g
Rhizoma seu Radix Notopterygii	10 g
Rhizoma Alismatis	10 g
Exocarpium Citri Grandis	6 g
Radix Glycyrrhizae	3 g
Succus Zingiberis	3 *spoonfuls*
Succus Bambusae	3 *spoonfuls*

EFFICACY

Strengthening the spleen, eliminating dampness, expelling wind, dissipating phlegm, relieving rheumatism and alleviating pain; mainly for cases of rheumatism manifested as localized arthralgia which will be aggravated in rainy days, fatigue, white and greasy fur on the tongue, wiry and smooth pulse, which are attributive to retention of dampness in the spleen and stomach and attack of wind-phlegm to the meridians and joints.

INDICATIONS

1. For cases of apoplexy manifested by distortion of the face, dysphasia, numbness and spasms of limbs, or even ehmiplegia, white and greasy fur on the tongue, wiry and smooth pulse, which are attributive to the attack of meridians by phlegm-dampness, omit Glycyrrhizae and add Scorpio, Bombyx Batrytica- tus.
2. For cases attributive to the attack of upper orifices by phlegm-dampness, which manifest as vertigo accompanied with nausea, vomiting, tinnitus,

deafness, white and greasy tongue fur and wiry pulse, add Rhizoma Pinelliae Praeparata, Rhizoma Gastrodiae and omit Glycyrrhizae.

3. Also applicable to cases with rheumatic arthritis, sciatica and beriberi attributive to accumulation of dmapness in the spleen and stomach; to cases of facial paralysis, poliomyelitis and thromboangiitis obliterans of cerebral bessels with hemiplesia attributive to attack of meridians by wind – phlegm; and to cases of hypertension and cerebral arteriosclerosis, with dizziness attributive to attack of the upper orifices by phlegm – dampness.

INTERPRETATION

Atractylodis acts as the chief drug in the prescription and is applied in large dosage, which has the effects of activating the spleen, drying dampness, eliminating wind and alleviating pain. Atractylodis Macrocephalae and Poria serve to strengthen the spleen and promote diuresis. Citri Grandis can regulate vital energy and acitivate the spleen, thus assists in eliminating dampness. Succus Zingiberis and Lophatheri are used to expel wind, dredge meridians and dissipate phlegm.

Decoction for Hemiplegia
(Xu Ming Tang)

INGREDIENTS

Lignum Cinnamomi	9 g
Radix Paeoniae Alba	9 g
Rhizoma Zingiberis	6 g
Herba Ephedrae	6 g
Rhizoma Ligustici Chuanxiong	6 g
Radix Codonopsis Pilosulae	6 g
Semen Armeniacae Amarum	6 g
Radix Angelicae Sinensis	9 g
Gypsum Fibrosum	15 g

Radix Glycyrrhizae   3 g

EFFICACY

Warming meridians, nourishing blood and expelling wind.

INDICATIONS

It is indicated for cases of hemiplegia after apoplexy, accompanied with weakness and rigidity of limbs, pale tongue with whitish fur, wiry and small pulse. Nowadays, it is usually applied for sequela of stroke. The action of this prescription is similar as that of the former, but its effect of warming meridians and strengthening yang energy is milder and has an additional effect of nourishing blood and expelling wind. It is suitable for cases of stroke attributive to deficiency of vital energy and blood and attack of the meridians by wind.

Decoction for Invigorating Spleen and Nourishing heart
(Gui Pi Tang)

INGREDIENTS

Radix Astragali seu Hedysari	15 g
Radix Codonopsis Pilosulae	15 g
Radix Angelicae Sinensis	12 g
Arillus Longan	12 g
Rhizoma Atractylodis Macrocephalae	10 g
Poria	10 g
Semen Ziziphi Spinosae	10 g
Radix Aucklandiae	5 g
Radix Glycyrrhizae Praeparata	5 g
Radix Polygalae	3 g
Rhizoma Zingiberis Recens	5 pcs

Fructus Ziziphi Jujubae   5 pcs

INDICATIONS

Benefiting vital energy, strengthening spleen, invigorating the heart and nourishing blood; mainly for cases due to hypofunction of heart and spleen and insufficiency of vital energy and blood, manifested as palpitation, amnesia, insomnia, fatigue poor appetite, sallow complexion, or preceded menstrual cycle with profuse pale or continuously dripping discharge, pale tongue with whitish fur, small and weak pulse. For cases of metrorrhagia attributive to failure of the spleen to control blood, subtract Aucklandiae and polygalae and add Fructus Corni to nourish liver and stop metrorrhagia. For case with hematochezia attributive to hypofunction of spleen with retention of cold evil, subtract Polygalae and add Zingiberis Praeparata to warm middle jiao and stopping bleeding. Also applicable to cases of pepticulcer, dysfunctional uterine bleeding, thrombocytopenia purpura, aplastic anemia etc. with hemorrhage attributive to hypofunction of heart and spleen.

INTERPRETATION

Astragali seu Hedysari and Codonopsis Pilosulae benefit vital energy and invigorate the spleen and serve as the chief drugs. Angelicae Sinensis and Arillus Longan tonify the blood, nourish the heart. The above four drugs used together strengthen both the heart and the spleen, and dealt with the primary aspect of the disease. Poria, Polygalae, Ziziphi Spinosae have the effects of nourishing the heart and calming the mental state, and dealt with the secondary aspect of the disease. Aucklandiae adn Atractylodis Macrocephalae strengthen the spleen adn regulate vital energy. Glycyrrhizae, Zingiberis Recens and Ziziphi Jujubae reconcile the action of spleen and stomach and promote the production of vital energy and blood. In summary, this prescription aims at benefiting vital energy and tonifying blood, when one's vital energy is sufficient, the heart is well nourished, the symptoms subside.

Chapter Twenty-one

Decoction for Invigorating Yang
(Bu Yang Huan Wu Tang)

INGREDIENTS

Radix Astragali seu Hedysari	60 g
Radix Angelicae Sinensis	15 g
Radix Paeoniae Rubra	15 g
Lumbricus	10 g
Rhizoma Ligustici Chuanxiong	10 g
Semen Persicae	6 g
Flos Carthami	6 g

EFFICACY

tonifying vital energy, promoting blood circulation and dredging the meridian passage; mainly for stroke sequelae such as hemiplegia, facial deviation, aphasia, slobbering, lower limbs paralyses, incontinence of urine, etc. with white fur and slow pulse.

INDICATIONS

1. For cases of unconsciousness attributed to sthenia-syndrome, the therapy for waking up from unconsciousness should be applied before the prescription is given.

2. The purpose of using crude sample of Astragali seu Hedysari is to remove blood stasis, therefore, a large dosage (beginning from 30 - 60 g should be applied in order to let it distributing all over the whole body.

3. For cases with much phlegm, add Rhizoma Arisaemacum Bile and Concretio Silicae Bambusae to eliminate the wind-phlegm; while for cases of aphasia, add Rhizoma Acori Graminei and Radix Polygalae to wake up the patient adn eliminate phlegm.

4. For cases of bi-syndrome due to deficiency of vital energy and blood sta-

sis, add Ramulus Taxilli to nourish the blood and eliminate wind evil.

5. The prescription may also be applicable to hemiplegia paraplegia, monoplegia resulting from cerebrovascular accidents and infantile paralysis, and rheumatic arthritis, rheumatoid arthritis, etc. attributed to deficiency of vital energy and blood stasis.

INTERPRETATION

Astragali seu Hedysari is the principal drug in this prescription, while has the effect of tonifying vital energy to promote blood circulation. The other ingredients have the effects of promoting blood circulation and dredging the meridiean passage. The prescription, as a whole, can tonify vital energy and also promote blood circulation, remove blood stasis but not hurt the healthy energy. When the vital energy is sufficient, the blood flow activated, the blood stasis is removed and the meridian passage is dredged, all the above – metioned disorders will be relieved.

Decoction for Mild Hemiplegia
(Xiao Xu Ming Tang)

INGREDIENTS

Lignum Cinnamomi	9 g
Radix Aconiti Praeparata	9 g
Radix Paeoniae Alba	9 g
Radix Ledebouriellae	9 g
Rhizoma zingiberis Recens	9 g
Herba Ephedrae	6 g
Rhizoma Ligustici Chuanxiong	6 g
Radix Codonopsis Pilosulae	6 g
Semen Armeniacae Amarum	6 g
Radix Scutellariae	6 g
Radix Stephaniae Tetrandrae	6 g

Chapter Twenty-one

Radix Glycyrrhizae   3 g

EFFICACY

Warming meridians, promoting the motion of yang-energy, supporting healthy energy and eliminating wind; mainly for cases of hemiplegia accompanied with distortion of the face, aphasia, spasm of limbs, headache, rigid neck, whitish fur on the tongue, tense pulse, which are attributive to deficiency of healthy energy and attack of wind-cold to meridians.

INDICATIONS

1. Applicable to rheumatism of wind-cold-dampness type with insufficiency of yang-energy, which manifests as wandering arthralgia, numbness of muscles and skin, limited movement of joints, white and smooth fur on the tongue, wiry and tense pulse.

2. This prescription is only suitable for stroke due to attack of the meridians by exogenous wind but contraindicated for cases of hemiplegia with distortion of the face of loss of consciousness which are attributive to impairment of liver and kidney, and the attack of asthenic wind inside the body.

3. Also applicable to cases of cerebral thrombosis and periodic paralysis with hemiplegia attributive to attack of meridians by wind-cold and to cases of chronic gouty arthritis, rheumatoid spondylitis, hyperplastic arthritis, etc. with arthralgia attributive to insufficiency of yang-energy and the attack of exogenous wind-cold-dampness.

INTERPRETATION

Ephedrae, ledebouriellae, Ligustic Chuanxiong and Armeniacae Amarum have the effects of dispelling superficial evils and warming and dredging meridians. Cinnamomi, Paeoniae Alba, Zingiberis Recens and Glycyrrhizae can regulate ying and wei, and not only enhance the effects of the above drugs but also increase the body resistance to defend against the attack of wind. Codonopsis Pilosulae and Aconiti Praeparata are used for benefiting vital energy and blood to restore the healthy energy and eliminate the evils when used with Paeoniae Alba and Ligustici Chuanxiong. Stephaniae Tetrandrae and Scutellariae can clear away the superficial heat and expel wind. Originally, there was Lignum Cinnamomi in the prescription, but it was often replaced by Ramulus Cinnamomi in the clinic. The former is good for warming the kidney to support yang, while the latter is for expelling wind, promoting sweating and warming and dredging the meridians. They may be applied accordingly.

Decoction for Removing Blood Stasis in the Chest
(Xue Fu Zhu Yu Tang)

INGREDIENTS

Radix Angelicae Sinensis	9 g
Rhizoma Ligustici Chuanxiong	5 g
Radix Paeoniae Rubra	9 g
Semen Persicae	12 g
Flos Carthami	9 g
Radix Bupleuri	3 g
Radix Platycodi	5 g
Fructus Aurantii	6 g
Radix Rehmanniae	9 g
Radix Glycyrrhizae	3 g
Radix Achyranthis Bidentatae	9 g

All the above drugs are to be decocted in water for oral administration.

EFFICACY

Promoting blood circulation to remove blood stasis and promoting circulation of qi to relieve pain.

INDICATIONS

1. Syndrome of blood stasis in the chest marked by long-standing prickly chest pain and headache which exist in a certain region, or endless hiccup, dysphoria due to interior heat, palpitation, insomnia, irritability and liability to a fit of temper, running a fever gradually at dusk, deep-red tongue with ecchymoses, dark-purple lips or dark eyes, uneven pulse or taut and tense pulse. Coronary heart disease, cerebral thrombosis, thromboangiitis, obliterans, hypertension, cirrhosis of liver, dysmenorrhea, amenia, headache, chest pain and hypochondriac pain marked by stagnancy of qi and blood stasis can be treated by the modified recipe.

INTERPRETATION

The leading ingredients in the recipe are Radix Angelicae Sinensis, Rhizoma Ligustici Chuanxiong, Radix Paeoniae Rubra, Semen Persicae, Flos Carthami and Radix Bupleuri, which promote blood circulation to remove blood stasis. Among them, Radix Bupleuri also ensures proper downward flow of the blood. Radix Platycodi soothes the liver and regulates the circulation of qi. Fructus Aurantii and Radix Rehmanniae relieve the oppressed feeling in the chest, promote the circulation of qi to render blood circulation to be normal. Radix Achyranthis Bidentatae removes heat from the blood and combines Radix Angelicae Sinensis to enrich the blood and moisten dryness so as to remove blood stasis without impairment of yin. Radix Glycyrrhizae cooridinates the effects of all the other ingredients in the recipe. Modern researches have proved that this recipe is especially effective in anti-coagulation and antispasm. Besides, it has some effect on uterine contraction.

CAUTIONS

1. Since this recipe is mainly composed of drugs for removing blood stasis, it should not be used to treat the syndrome without distinct stasis.
2. Contraindicated for pregnant cases.

Decoction for Sterility
(Hua Shui Zhong Zi Tang)

INGREDIENTS

Radix Morindae Officinalis (*soaked in salt solution*)	10 g
Poria	10 g
Radix Codonopsis Pilosulae	10 g
Semen Cuscutae (*fried with wine*)	10 g
Semen Euryales (*fried*)	10 g
Rhizoma Atractylodis Macrocephalae (*fried with earth*)	12 g
Semen Plantaginis (*fried with wine*)	6 g
Cortex Cinnamomi	2 g

EFFICACY

Warming the kidney, strengthening the spleen and promoting diuresis, mainly for cases of sterility accompanied with lumbago, aversion to cold, cold limbs, fatigue, flat taste in the mouth, poor appetite, oliguria, edema of the lower limbs, puffiness of the body, corpulent tongue with white and greasy fur, sunken and slow pulse, which are attributive to deficiency of spleen - yang and kidney - yang, and retention of dampness in the uterus.

INDICATIONS

1. Applicable to cases of impotence or nocturnal emission accompanied with dizziness, spiritlessness, lumbago, weakness of lower limbs, pale complexion, poor appetite, loose stools, pale tongue with white fur, sunken and slow pulse, which are attributive to declination of life - gate fire and deficiency of kidney - qi.

2. Also indicated for cases with general pitted edema which is more prominent in the lower part, lumbago, fatigue, cold limbs, aversion to cold, oliguria, poor appetite, loose stools, corpulent tongue with white smooth fur, sunken and slow pulse, which are attributive to deficiency of spleen - yang and kidney - yang

and accumulation of cold-dampness in the interior.

3. Also applicable to cases of endocrine disorder such as hypothyroidism, and pelvic diseases such as endometritis with sterility attributive to deficiency of spleen-yang and retention of dampness in the uterus; to cases of hypogonadism and neurasthenia with impotence or nocturnal emission attributive to the declination of life-gate fire and deficiency of kidney-qi; and to cases of chronic nephritis with edema attributive to deficiency of spleen-yang and kidney-yang and accumulation of cold-dampness in the interior.

Decoction for Treating Rheumatism
(Juan Bi Tang)

INGREDIENTS

Rhizoma seu Radix Notopterygii	10 g
Rhizoma Curcumae Longae	10 g
Radix Angelicae Sinensis (soaked with wine)	10 g
Radix Paeoniae Alba	10 g
Radix Ledebouriellae	10 g
Radix Astragalae seu hedysari	15 g
Radix Glycyrrhizae Praeparata	6 g
Rhizoma Zingiberis Recens	5 pcs

EFFICACY

Expelling wind and dampness, benefiting vital energy and nourishing blood; mainly for rheumatism of wind type attributive to the stagnation of wind-cold-dampness evil (predominantly the wind evil) in the meridians, which is manifested as immobility of the joints, wandering arthralgia, especially the neck, back, shoulder and elbow, thin and white fur on the tongue, floating and slow pulse.

INDICATIONS

1. Applicable to cases of stroke manifested by deviation of the eyes and mouth, numbness of the muscles and skin, spasm of limbs, or hemiplegia (especially the upper limb), thin and whitish fur on the tongue, floating and wiry pulse, which are attributive to weakness of the superficies, deficiency of vital energy and attack of wind evil.

2. Also applicable to cases of rheumatic arthritis, rheumtoid arthritis, facial paralysis, cerebral accidents, etc., which are attributive to the stagnation of wind – cold – dampness evil (predominantly the wind evil) in the meridians.

INTERPRETATION

Nontopterygii and Ledebouriellae can expel wind evil, remove dampness evil and relieve pain, and is especially suitable for rheumatism of the upper body. Astragali seu Heday sari and Glycyrrhizae Praeparata have the effects of supp0lementing vital energy and strengthening the body surface and is helpful for expelling wind evil. Meanwhile, Astragali seu Heday sari and Glycyrrhizae Praeparata exert a tonifying effect without causing indigestion, and Notopterygii and Ledebouriellae promote vital energy circulation without losing it when all are used together. Angelicae Sinensis and Paeoniae Alba can nourish blood and promote blood circulation, Curcumae Longae is used for regulating vital energy in the blood; they are applied together for nourishing the blood to eliminate wind. Zingiberis Recens helps Notopterygii and Ledebouriellae to expel wind and dampness, and also helps Astragali seu Hedysari and Glycyrrhizae Praeparata to cooridinate ying – qi and wei – qi. Therefore, the prescription is also suitable for bi – syndrome due to wind – cold – dampness evil, characterized by deficiency of both ying – qi and wei – qi.

Decoction of Bupleuri Adding Os Draconis and Concha Ostreae
(Chaihu Jia Longgu Muli Tang)

INGREDIENTS

Radix Bupleuri	10 g
Radix Sutellariae	6 g
Rhizoma zingiberis Recens	6 g
Radix Codonopsis Pilosulae	6 g
Ramulus Cinnamomi	6 g
Radix et Rhizoma Rhei	6 g
Poria	6 g
Rhizoma Pinelliae	6 g
Minium	1 g
Fructus Ziziphi Jujubae	3 pcs
Os Draconis	15 g
Concha Ostreae	15 g

EFFICACY

Regulating shaoyang, dispersing phlegm, tranquilizing, supporting healthy energy and eliminating evil; mainly for cases attributive to invasion of heat to shaoyang (liver and gallbladder), which manifest feeling of oppression over the chest and hypochondrium, restlessness, delirium, frightening, insomnia, fatigue, red tongue with yellow fur, wiry and rapid pulse, i.e., the simultaneous occurence of asthenia - and sthenia - syndrome, cold = and heat - syndrome, as well as superficies - and interior - syndrome.

INDICATIONS

1. Minium is a poinsonous drug and should not be taken more than 10 g at one time and not for a long period. Now it is usually replaced by Ferrum scale.
2. Applicable to cases of epilepsy accom = panied with dizziness, fatigue,

pale complexion, red tongue with white and greasy fur, wiry and smooth pulse, which are attributive to adverse rising of wind – phlegm with simultaneous occurence of asthenia – and sthenia – syndrome.

3. Also indicated for cases of tinnitus and deafness accompanied with profuse expectoration, bitter taste in the mouth, feeling of oppression over the chest and hypochondrium, dizziness, fatigue, red tongue with yellow fur, wiry and rapid pulse, which are attributive to the adverse rising of phlegm – fire from the liver and gallbladder, with simultaneous occurence of asthenia – and sthenia – syndrome.

4. Also applicable to cases of hyperthyroidism, schizophrenia and neurasthenia marked by palpitation, which are attributive to the invasion of heat to shaoyang (liver and gallbladder); and to cases of Meniere's syndrome and sequelae of cerebral concussion marked by tinnitus and dizziness, which are attributive to adverse rising of phlegm – fire from the liver, gallbladder, with simultaneous occurrence of asthenia – and sthenia – syndrome.

INTERPRETATION

The prescription is composed on the basis of the Decoction of Bupleuri for Regulating Shaoyang, by adding Ramulus Cinnamomi, Rhei, Poria, Minium, Os Draconis, Concha Ostreae and omitting Glycyrrhizae from it. Bupleuri serves to eliminate the pathogens from the interior when it is used together with Ramulus Cinnamomi and to clear away the heat located between the superificies and the interior when it is used together with Scutellariae. Rhei can directly clear away the interior heat. Pinelliae, Zingiberis Recens and Minium disperse phlegm and eliminate accumulated heat. Os Draconis and Concha Ostreae act as sedative. Codonopsis Pilosulae, Ziziphi Jujubae and Poria are applied for strengthening the spleen, benefiting vital energy and supporting healthy energy. In sum, the prescription aims at eliminating pathogens both from the superificies and interior by applying drugs both cold and warm in ntaure, tonifying and purging as well as descending and ascending in action.

Chapter Twenty-one

Decoction of Bupleuri and Puerariae for Expelling Evil from Musices (Chai Ge Jie Ji Tang)

INGREDIENTS

Radix Bupleuri	10 g
Radix Puerariae	10 g
Gypsum Fibrosum	10 g
Radix Scutellariae	6 g
Radix Paeoniae Lactiflorae	6 g
Rhizoma seu Radix Notopterygii	6 g
Radix Angelicae Dahuriae	6 g
Radix Glycyrrhizae	3 g
Radix Platycodi	3 g
Rhizoma Zingiberis Recens	3 pcs
Fructus Ziziphi Jujubae	3 pcs

EFFICACY

Expelling the evil from the superficies, lowering fever and clearing away the interior heat evil; mainly for common cold of wind-cold type with formation of heat, which is manifested by chilliness becoming milder and fever higher, headache, soreness of limbs, eyes pain, thin and yellowish fur on the tongue, floating and bounding pulse, etc..

INDICATIONS

1. For cases of warm-type malaria manifested by high fever, mild chilliness, general aching, red tongue with yellowish fur, wiry and rapid pulse, omit Radix Glycyrrhizae and Radix Platycodi and add Fructus Tsaoko eliminate dampness.

2. For cases of heat-type arthralgia manifested by joint aching, fever, chilliness, yellowish and greasy fur on the tongue, omit Radix Glycyrrhizae and Radix Platycodi, and add Cortex Phellodendri and Ramulus Cinnamomi to elimi-

nate dampness–heat, dredge the meridians and relieve pain.

3. Applicable to cases of wind–fire toothache manifested by toothache referring to the head, chilliness, red tongue with whitish fur, wiry pulse.

4. Also applicable to cases of influenza, trigeminal neuralgia, rheumatic arthritis, etc. which are attributive to heat formation by stagnation of cold.

INTERPRETATION

Bupleuri and Puerariae have the effects of expelling the evil from the superficies and lowering fever. Notopterygii and Angelica Dahuricae have the effect of expelling wind evil from the body surface. Scutellariae and Gypsum Fibrosum have the effect of clearing away the interior heat evil. Paeoniae Lactiflorae is helpful to regulate ying and clear away heat evil. Platycodi helps Bupleuri to expel evil. Zingiberis Recens, Ziziphi Jujubae and Glycyrrhizae regulate the function of ying and wei and then the middle jiao. Although this prescription composes of the drugs of cold nature as well as those of warm nature, but, as a whole, its cold nature is greater than warm nature. However, it is still a prescription of acrid flavour and cool nature, which expels wind–heat.

Decoction of Cimicifugae and Astragali seu Hedysari
(Shengma Huangqi Tang)

INGREDIENTS

Radix Astragali seu Hedysari	30 g
Radix Angelicae Sinensis	12 g
Rhizoma Cimicifugae	6 g
Radix Bupleuri	6 g

EFFICACY

Benefiting vital energy, lifting yang and activating vital energy; mainly for cases of dysuria attributive to dysfunction of vital energy, which manifest difficult and dripping urination, tiredness, shortness of breath, pale tongue, slow and weak pulse.

INDICATIONS

1. For cases attributing to deficiency and collapes of vital energy and downward flowing of essential substance, which manifest prolonged discharge of rice-water like urine, pale complexion, fatigue, pale tongue and feeble pulse, add Fructus Corni to keep the essential substance.

2. for protracted cases of nocturnal emission or enuresis accompanied with listlessness, pale complexion, pale tongue, sunken and feeble pulse, which are attributive to deficiency of vital energy, add Fructus Schisandrae and Ootheca Mantidis to calm the mental state and astringe the essential substance (or urine).

3. Also applicable to cases of chronic prostatitis, neurasthenia, senile dementia, etc. with difficult urination or enuresis, which are attributive to dysfunction of vital energy.

INTERPRETATION

This prescription is developed from the Decoction for Strengthening Middle Jiao and Benefiting Qi which is mainly for collapse of middle-jiao energy and hypofunction of spleen and stomach. In the prescription, Astragalic seu Hedysari is applied together with Cimicifugae for supplementing vital energy and raising yang to restore with Cimicifugae for supplementing vital energy and raising yang to restore the normal function of vital energy. Angelicae Sinensis and Bupleuri can disperse the stagnated liver-energy. In sum, the purpose of this prescription is to lift up collapse vital energy and restore the normal urination.

Decoction of Cinnamomi Aconiti
(Guizhi Fuzi Tang)

INGREDIENTS

Ramulus Cinnamomi	12 g
Radix Aconiti Praeparata	10 g
Rhizoma Zingiberis Recens	10 g
Fructus Ziziphi Jujubae	8 pcs
Radix Glycyrrhizae Praeparata	6 g

EFFICACY

Expelling wind and dampness, warming meridians and eliminating cold; mainly for cases attributive to the attack of wind − cold − dampness to the muscles and meridians, and circulatory impediment of vital energy and blood, which manifest general aching, immovability of trunk and limbs, no thirst nor vomiting, white and greasy fur, floating and unsmooth pulse.

INDICATIONS

1. Applicable to cases with a yang − deficiency constitution and affection of wind − cold, which manifest chilliness, fever, aversion to wind, sweating, headache, cold limbs, tiredness of somnolence, white and greasy fur, sunken and slow pulse.

2. Also indicated for cases with chest apin referring to the back, feeling of oppression over the chest, tiredness, white and greasy fur on the tongue, wiry and slow pulse, which are attributive to accumulation of cold − dampness.

3. Also applicable to cases of rheumatic arthritis, sciatic periomarthritis, etc. with chillness and fever attributive to yang − deficiency and affection of exogenous wind − cold; and to cases of emphysema, coronary heart disease, rheumatic heart disease, etc. with chest pain attributive to accumulation of wind − phlegm.

INTERPRETATION

Aconiti has the effects of warming the meridians and eliminating cold - dmapness from the meridians. They two act as the principal drugs of the prescription. Zingiberis Recens and Ziziphi Jujubae serve to regulate ying and wei and can warm the meridians and promote the circulation of vital energy and blood when they are used together with Cinnamomi.

Decoction of Cinnamomi, Glycyrrhizae, etc.
(Guizhi Gancao Longgu Muli Tang)

INGREDIENTS

Ramulus Cinnamomi	10 g
Radix Clycyrrhizae Praeparata	15 g
Os Draconis	30 g
Concha Ostreae	30 g

EFFICACY

Warming heart - yang energy and tranquilizing; mainly for cases attributive to impairment of heart - yang, which manifest palpitation, irritability, spontaneous sweating, pale tongue with white and greasy fur, floating and slow, or slow pulse with irregular intervals.

INDICATIONS

1. For cases attributive to severe deficiency of heart - yang, which manifest sweating, cold limbs, feeble and large or slow and weak pulse, add Radix Aconiti Praeparata to recuperate the depleted yang.

2. Applicable to cases of nocturnal emission with dizziness, fatigue, spiritlessness, reddish tongue, small and slow pulse, which are attributive to ineqilibri-

um between yin and yang.

3. Also applicable to cases of rheumatic heart disease, sinus bradycardia and atrioventricular block with palpitation, which are attributive to deficiency of heart − yang; and to cases of neurasthenia and hypogonadism with nocturnal emission, which are attributed to inequilibrium of yin and yang.

INTERPRETATION

Glycyrrhizae is used in a large dose in this prescription and serves particulary to relieve palpitation and irritability. In sum, this prescription aims chiefly at warming and promoting heart − yang. Palpitation and other symptoms mentioned above may subside when the heart − yang is restored.

Decoction of Cinnamomi, Paeoniae and Aemarrhenae
(Guizhi Shaoyao Zhimu Tang)

INGREDIENTS

Ramulus Cinnamomi	10 g
Radix Paeoniae Alba	10 g
Rhizoma Zingiberis Recens	10 g
Rhizoma Atractylodis Macrocephalae	10 g
Radix Anemarrhenae	10 g
Radix Ledebouriellae	10 g
Radix Aconiti Praeparata	6 g
Herba Ephedrae	5 g
Radix Glycyrrhizae	3 g

EFFICACY

Expelling wind and dampness, activating yang − energy, relieving arthralgia, regulating yin and clearing away heat, mainly for cases with severe and imgratory arthralgia with swelling and increased temperature of the affected joints, dizzines, fatigue, nausea, vomiting, emaciation, thin and yellow greasy fur on the tongue, rapid pulse, which are attributive to accumulation of wind and dampness with production of heat evil.

INDICATIONS

1. This prescription is suitable for arthralgia of wind - dampness type with formation of heat. It is not indicated for those cases with severe heat which manifest high fever, thirst, red tongue with yellow and dry fur, smooth and rapid bounding pulse.

2. Applicable to cases of apoplexy involving the meridians manifested by hemiplegia, rigidity of limbs, dizziness, thin and yellow greasy fur on the tongue, wiry pulse, which are attributive to prolonged retention of wind and phlegm - dampness in the meridians with transformation of heat.

3. Also applicable to cases of chronic gouty arthritis, rheumatic arthritis, periomarthritis, etc. attributive to accumulation of wind - dampness with trnasformation of heat; and to cases of sequela of cerebrovascular accident and rheumatic cerebrobvasculitis with hemiplegia, which are attributive to retention of wind and phlegm - dampness in the meridians.

INTERPRETATION

Ramulus Cinnamomi, Ledebouriellae, Ephedrae and Atractylodis Macrocephalae are used together to eliminate wind - dampness from both superficies and interior. Paeoniae Alba and Anemarrhenae have the effects of regulating yin and clearing away heat. Aconiti serves to activate yang - energy, expel dampness and alleviate pain when it is used together with Ramulus Cinnamomi, Paeoniae Alba and Anemarrhenae. It is noteworthy that drugs of both hot and cold or yin and yang nature are used simultaneously in the prescription, and their actions are promoted each other instead of antagonized.

Antipyretic and Antitoxic Bolus
(Qingwen Jiedu Wan)

Ingredients

Folium Isatidis
Fructus Forsythiae
Radix Scrophulariae
Radix Trichosanthis
Radix Platycodi
Fructus Arctii
Radix Seu Rhizoma Notopterygii
Radix Angelicae Dahuricae
Radix Ledebouriellae
Radix Puerariae
Radix Scutellariae
Radix Bupleuri
Rhizoma Ligustici Chuanxiong
Radix Paeoniae Rubra
Radix Glycyrrhizae
Herba Lophatheri

Efficacy

Having antipyretic and antitoxic functions.
Honey boluses, 9 g each bolus; 10 boluses per box.

Indications

Influenza, marked by fever with chills, anhidrosis with headache, thirst and dry throat, aching pain of limbs. It is also used to treat swelling and pain of mumps.

Administration and Dosage

To be taken orally, one bolus each time, twice a day. For children, the doses should be correspondingly reduced.

Bolus of Calculus Bovis for Purging the Heart-Fire
(Niuhuang qingxin wan)

Ingredients

Calculus Bovis	0.75 g
Cinnabaris	4.5 g
Rhizoma Coptidis	15 g
Radix Scutellariae	9 g
Fructus Gardeniae	9 g
Radix Curcumae	6 g

Indications

Clearing away heat evil and toxic material, waking up patients from unconsciousness by eliminating phlegm; mainly for seasonal febrile diseases with heat evil involving the pericardium and the phlegm-heat evil stagnating in the heart, which are manifested by high fever, irritability, coma, delirium, red tongue with yellowish fur.

Bolus of Citri Grandis
(Juhe wan)

Ingredients

Semen Citri Grandis	30 g
Sargassum	10 g

Thallus Laminariae seu Eckloniae	10 g
Thallus Laminariae Japonicae	10 g
Fructus Meliae Toosendan	10 g
Cortex Magnoliae Officinalis	10 g
Semen Persicae	6 g
Caulis Akebiae	6 g
Radix Aucklandiae	6 g
Lignum Cinnamomi	3 g

Efficacy

Activating circulation of vital qi and blood, dredging the passage of yang-qi, promoting diuresis, dissolving phlegm and softening the hard lumps; mainly for swelling of scrotum due to phlegm-dampness, with pain referred to the abdomen, whitish and greasy fur on the tongue and wiry pulse.

Indications

1. This prescription is applicable to cases with persistent swelling of scrotum. For cases with severe pain, add *Radix Angelicae Sinensis* and *Radix Cyathulae* to eliminate blood stasis and relieving pain; for cases with cold pain, add *Fructus Foeniculi* and *Fructus Evodiae* to warm the liver and expel the cold evil. In cases of transformation to heat from cold-dampness with redness, swelling, itching or yellowish discharge over the scrotum and oliguria, subtract *Lignum Cinnamomi* and add *Cortex Phellodendri*, *Radix Gentianae*, to clear away heat and dampness.

2. For single or multiple, smooth, and painless goiters attributive to stagnation of vital qi and phlegm, subtract *Caulis Akebiae*, and *Meliae Toosendan* and add *Rhizoma Cyperi* and *Bulbus Fritillariae Thunbergii* to promote circulation of vital qi and eliminate phlegm.

3. For cases of breast nodules, unilateral or bilateral, round or oval, smooth or nodular, attributive to stagnation of vital qi and phlegm, subtract *Caulis Akebiae* and add *Fructus hordei Germinatus* (in a large dosage) and *Retinervus Citri Fructus* to disperse the depressed liver-qi and dissolving phlegm.

4. Also applicable to case of hydrocele of tunica vaginalis, varicocele of spermatic cord, thyroid adenoma, breast fibroadenoma, etc. attributive to stagnation of vital qi and phlegm.

Interpretation

Semen Citri Grandis, bitter in taste and warm in nature, is an agent for regulating vital qi, dispersing stagnation and relieving pain. *Meliae Toosendan*, *Aucklandiae*, *Aurantii Immaturus* and *Magnoliae Officinalis* have the effects of dispersing the depressed liver - qi, relieving pain and promoting diuresis. *Laminarriae seu Eckloniae*, *Sargassum* and *Laminariae japonicae* serve to soften hard lumps, dissolve phlegm and disperse stagnation. *Lignum Cinnamomi* together with *Persicae* and *Corydalis* can warm the meridians and activate blood circulation; while together with *Aucklandiae* can promote diuresis and lead the dampness downwards.

Bolus of Rhei and Eupolyphaga seu Steleophaga
(Dahuang zhechong wan)

Ingredients

Radix et Rhizoma Rhei (steamed)	8 g
Eupolyphaga seu Steleophaga	6 g
Radix Scutellariae	6 g
Radix Glycyrrhizae	6 g
Semen Persicae	6 g
Semen Armeniacae Amarum	6 g
Tabanus Bivittatus	6 g
Holotrichia Diomphalia	6 g
Radix Paeoniae Alba	12 g
Radix Rehmanniae	30 g
Dry Lacquer	3 g
Hirudo	8 set

Grind the above ingredients into powder and is prepared as boluses, taken with warm wine.

Efficacy

Eliminating blood stasis and masses, nourishing blood to promote tissue regeneration; mainly for consumptive diseases attributive to retention of blood stasis in the body, which are manifested by emaciation, abdominal fullness, anorexia, squamation and dryness of skin, blackish coloration around the eyes, petechiae on the tongue, wiry and unsmooth pulse, etc..

Indications

1. For cases with localized abdominal pain and tenderness, dry stools, dark purplish tongue, wiry and small, smooth pulse, which are attributive to stagnation of blood and vital energy, hyperactivity of evil and sthenia of healthy energy, the prescription may be used as an analgesic and blood-stasis eliminating agent.
2. Also indicated for cases of erysipelas of the leg with lymphangitis, dark reddish tongue, wiry and unsmooth pulse, which are attributive to obstruction of meridians by blood stasis and heat.
3. Applicable to cases of amenorrhea accompanied with localized aching and marked tenderness over the lower abdomen, emaciation, purplish spots at the margin of the tongue, wiry and small, unsmooth pulse, which are attibutive to the stagnation of liver-blood.
4. Also applicable to cases of cirrhosis of liver, pulmonary tuberculosis, gastric cancer, thrombophlebitis, osteomyelitis, etc., which are attributive to retention of blood stasis in the body or obstruction of the meridians by blood stasis and heat.

Interpretation

Rhei activates blood circulation and eliminates blood stasis; *Eupolyphaga seu Steleophaga* removes stagnated blood and eliminates masses. They act together to discharge the blood stasis with feces. *Tabanus Bivittatus*, *Holotrichia*

Diomphalia, *Lacquer*, *Persicae* and *Hirudo* are applied to activate blood circulation and dredge the passage of meridians, and also applied № 6 to open the stagnated lung-qi and promote blood circulation; they all serve to increase the effect of eliminating blood stasis. № 10, 9 and № 4 can nourish blood and vessels to support healthy energy. № 3 purges stagnancy-heat which may be formed by blood stasis. Wine serves to enhance the effect of other drugs.

Bolus of Six Drugs Including Rehmannia
(Liuwei dihuang wan)

Ingredients

Rhizoma Rehmanniae Praeparata	240 g
Fructus Corni	120 g
Rhizoma Dioscoreae	120 g
Rhizoma Alismatis	90 g
Poria	90 g
Cortex Moutan Radicis	90 g

Grind the drugs into fine powder and mix with honey to make boluses as big as the seed of *Chinese parasol*, to be administered orally 6-9 grams each time with warm boiled water or slight salt water, twice or three times a day. The drugs can also be decocted in water for oral administration with the dosage reduced in proportion as the original recipe.

Efficacy

Nourishing and enriching the liver and kidney.

Indications

Syndrome due to the deficiency of vital esence of liver and kidney with symptoms of weakness and soreness of waist and knees, vertigo, tinnitus, deafness, night sweat, emission as well as persistant opening of fontanel. Or the flaring up of sthenic fire resulting in symptoms such as hectic fever, feverish sensation in the palms and soles, diabetes or toothache due to fire of deficiency type, dry mouth and throat, red tongue with little fur, and thready and rapid pusle.

Since it tends to be greasy tonics, the recipe should be administered carefully to patients with weakened function of the spleen in transporting and distributing nutrients and water.

In addition, the above recipe can be modified to treat many other disease indicating the syndrome due to the deficiency of vital essence of liver and kidney such as vegetative nerve functional disturbance, hypertension, arteriosclerosis, diabetes, chronic nephritis, hyperthyroidism, pulmonary tuberculosis, chronic urinary infection, bronchial asthma, amenorrhea, scanty menstruation, or infantile dysplasia and interlectual hypoevolutism.

Interpretation

Prepared *rhizome of rehmannia*, as the principal one, possesses the effect of nourishing the kidney - yin and supplementing the essence of life. As assistant drugs, *dogwood fruit*, sour in flavor and warm in nature, is used for nourishing the kidney and replenishing the liver, while dried *Chinese yam* for nourishing the kidney - yin and tonifying the spleen. The rest ingredients collectively play the role of adjuvant drus. *Oriental water plantain* coordinates with the principal drug in clearing the kidney and purging turbid evils, *moutan bark* cooperates with dogwood fruit in purging liver fire, and poria shares the effort together with dried *Chinese yam* to excrete dampness from the spleen. The whole recipe acts as both tonics and purgatives with tonifying effect dominant.

Clinically and experimentally, the recipe has the effects of nourishing the body and consolidating the constitution, inhibiting hypercatabolism, reducing excitement of the brain, adjusting endocrine function and vegetative nerve, lowering blood pressure and blood sugar, inducing diuresis, improving the function of the kidney as well as promoting the epithelial hyperplasia of the esophagus and preventing cancer, etc..

Bolus of Ten Powerful Tonics
(Shiquan dabu wan)

Ingredients

Radix Codonopsis Pilosulae
Rhizoma Atractylodis Macrocephalae
Poria
Radix Glycyrrhizae
Radix Angelicae Sinensis
Rhizoma Ligustici Chuanxiong
Radix Paeoniae Alba
Radix Rehmanniae Praeparata
Radix Astragali seu Hedysari
Cortex Cinnamomi

Honeyed boluses, 9 g each bolus, 10 boluses per box. To be taken orally, one bolus each time, twice or three times daily.

Efficacy

Warming and nourishing qi and blood.

Indications

Deficiency of both qi and blood marked by sallow complexion, short breath, palpitation, dizziness, spontaneous perspiration, mental fatigue, lassitude of the extremities, profuse menstruation. It also serves as a supporting drug to detoxicating drugs in the treatment of non-healing of ulcers due to deficiency of qi and blood.

Cow-bezoar Bolus for Clearing Away Heat of the Upper Part of the Body
(Niuhuang shang qing wan)

Ingredients

Calculus Bovis
Herba Menthae
Flos Schizonepetae
Radix Ligustici Chuanxiong
Fructus Gardeniae
Rhizoma Coptidis
Cortex Phellodendri
Radix Scutellariae
Radix et Rhizoma Rhei
Fructus Forsythiae
Radix Paeoniae Rubra
Radix Angelicae Sinensis
Radix Rehmanniae
Radix Platycodi
Gypsum Fibrosum
Borneolum
Radix Glycyrrhizae

Grind the above drugs into fine powder, mix it with honey and make them into boluses, 6 g each bolus, 10 boluses per box.

Administration and Dosage

To be taken orally, one bolus each time, twice a day.

Efficacy

Clearing away heat and purging pathogenic fire, dispelling wind and relieving pain.

Indications

The syndromes of excessive fire in the middle and upper parts of the human body or the attack of pathogenic wind and heat on the upper part of the body marked by headache, vertigo, conjunctival congestion, tinnitus, swelling and sore throat, ulcerations of the mouth and tongue, swelling and soreness of the gums, constipation and dry stool.

Cautions

Pregnant women should be careful when taking this medicine.

Decoction for Clearing Away Pestilent Factors and Detoxification
(Qingwen baidu yin)

Ingredients

Cornu Rhinocerotis	18 – 24 g; 9 – 15 g; 6 – 12 g
Rhizoma Coptidis	12 – 18 g; 6 – 12 g; 3 – 5 g
Fructus Gardeniae	6 – 9 g
Radix Platycodi	6 – 9 g
Radix Scutellariae	6 – 9 g
Rhizoma Anemarrhenae	6 – 9 g
Radix Paeoniae Rubra	6 – 9 g
Radix Scrophulariae	6 – 9 g
Fructus Forsythiae	6 – 9 g
Radix Glycyrrhizae	6 – 9 g
Cortex Moutan Radicis	6 – 9 g
Herba Lophatheri	6 – 9 g

Efficacy

Clearing away heat evil and toxic materials, cooling blood and supporting yin; mainly fro cases of seasonal epidemic diseses attributive to hyperactivity of severe heat in qifen and xuefen, which are manifested by high fever, restlessness, or even mania and delirium, thirst, intense headache, purplish red eruptions, hematemesis, epistaxis, dry lips, crimson tongue, rapid pulse.

Indications

1. The prescription is widely applicable to cases of internal medicine and surgery.

2. For critical cases of furunculosis complicated by septicemia attributive to the attack of viscera by toxic material, add *Flos Lonicerae* and omit *Lophatheri* and *Scrophulariae*.

3. For cases with general aching, intense headache, lumbago, oliguria, high fever, irritability, which are attributive to the attack of fire and pestilent evil, omit *Platycodi* and *Glycyrrhizae* and add *Rhizoma Imperatae* to nourish yin and promote diuresis. Nowadays, it is also applied for cases of leptospirosis with the above symptoms.

4. For cases with discharge of fresh or darkish bloody stools, high fever, irritability, red tongue, dry lips, sunken and small, rapid pulse, which are attributive to severe attack of pestilent evil, omit *Glycyrrhizae*, *Platycodi*, *Lophatheri*, *Forsythiae* and add *Flos Carthami*. Nowadays, it is also applied for cases of necrotizing enterocolitis with the same mechanism.

5. Also applicable to epidmeic meningitis, scarlet fever, erysipelas of face, septicemia, etc. attributive to the attack of pestilent evil and hyperactivity of heat in qifen and xuefen.

Interpretation

This prescription is composed of the modificatins of *White tiger decoction*, *Decoction of Coptidis for Detoxification* and *Decoction of Cornu Rhioncerotis and Rehmanniae*. *Gypsum Fibrosum*, *Anemarrhenae*, *Glycyrrhizae* and

Lophatheri have the effect of clearing away sthenic heat in qifen. *Coptidis*, *Gardeniae*, *Scutellariae* and *Forsythiae* have the effects of puring fire and elimination toxic materials. *Cornu Rhinocerotis*, *Rehmanniae*, *Moutan Radicis*, *Paeoniae Rubra* and *Scrophulariae* have the effects of cooling blood and preserving ying. The combination of three prescriptions constituents a strong agent for clearing away heat evil and toxic material.

Decoction for Clearing Heat in Ying System
(Qing ying tang)

Ingredients

Cornu Rhinocerotis	2 g
Radix Rehmanniae	15 g
Radix Scrophulariae	9 g
Herba Lophatheri	3 g
Radix Ophiopogonis	9 g
Radix Salviae Miltiorrhizae	6 g
Rhizoma Coptidis	5 g
Flos Lonicerae	9 g
Fructus Forsythiae	6 g

All the above drugs are to be decocted in water for oral administration.

Efficacy

Clearing and dispelling pathogenic heat from ying system, nourishing yin and promoting blood circulation.

Indications

Invasion of ying system by pathogenic heat manifested by feverish body which is aggravated in the night, delirium, insomnia due to vexation, or by faint skin rashes, deep-red and dry tongue and rapid pulse.

The recipe can also be modified to deal with ying-syndrome occuring in epidemic encephalitis B, epidemic cerebrospinal meningitis, septicemia and other infectious diseases.

Interpretation

In the recipe, *Cornu Rhinocerotis*, being salty in flavour and cold in property, and *Radix Rehmanniae* being sweet in taste and cold in nature, both exert a role of a principal drug, having the effect of removing heat from ying and blood systems. *Scrophulariae* and *Ophiopogonis* together act as assistant drugs having the effect of nourishing yin and clearing heat. The rest share the role of adjuvant and guiding drugs. *Lophatheri*, *Ophiopogonis*, *Lonicerae* and *Forsythiae* are used to clear and dispel pathogenic heat from ying system through qi system, and *Salviae Miltiorrhizae* is used to promote blood circulation to remove blood stasis.

Clinically and Experimentally, it is ascertained that the recipe possesses the efficacies of relieving inflammation, bringing down fever, tranquilizing the mind, resisting bacteria and viruses, tonifying the heart, arresting bleeding improving immunologic function, promoting blood circulation and so on.

Cases with white and slippery coating of the tongue which suggests invasion by pathogenic dampness should not use recipe in case it encourages pathogenic dampness.

Decoction for Strngthening Middle Jiao and Benefiting Vital Energy
(Bu zhong yi qi tang)

Ingredients

Radix Astragali seu Hedysari	15 g
Radix Codonopsis Pilosulae	15 g
Radix Angelicae Sinensis	10 g
Rhizoma Atractylodis Macrodephalae	10 g
Exocarpium Citri Grandis	6 g
Radix Glycyrrhizae Praeparata	6 g

Rhizoma Cimicifugae	3 g
Radix Bupleuri	3 g
Fructus Ziziphi Jujubae	6 g
Rhizoma Zingiberis Recens	6 g

Decoct the above ingredients in a right amount of water for oral administration.

Efficacy

Strengthening spleen, benefiting qi, lifting up yang - qi, mainly for the cases with deficiency of spleen and stomach and collapse of middle - jiao energy, manifested by shortness of breath, disinclination for speaking, tiredness, weakness, or prolapse of rectum, or fever due to deficiency of qi, pale tongue with white fur, empty and weak pulse.

Indications

1. This prescription is originally applied to fever due to internal damage, and now commonly for prolapse of rectum, gastroptosis and prolapse of uterus due to deficiency and collapse of qi.

2. Applicable to cases of common cold with deficiency of qi manifesting lingering fever, profuse sweating, pale tongue and weak pulse.

3. Also applicable to cases of septicemia, pulmonary tuberculosis, aplastic anemia, leukemia and summer fever which are manifested by fever due to deficiency of qi.

Interpretation

Astragali seu Hedysari has the effects of tonifying and lifting up qi; № 2, 4 and № 6 have the effects of strengthening the spleen and regulating the stomach, helping № 1 to tonify qi. While № 7 and № 8 have the effects of leading the stomach - qi upward, helping № 1 to lift up qi. № 3 can nourish blood and help qi to flow toward its bases. The case with deficiency of qi usually suffers from stagnation of qi, so the prescription includes № 5, 10 and № 9 to regulate qi and the stomach.

Modern studies have confirmed that the recipe has the efficacies in improving the cellular immune function promoting metabolism, improving the excitement of cerebral cortex, promoting the tension of skeletal muscles, smooth muscles and supporting tissues; and promoting digestion and absorption.

Cautions

Patients with internal heat due to yin deficiency is prohibited from taking this recipe, and for those with the impairment of body fluid and qi after illness, it's better to prescribe this recipe together with other drugs.

Decoction of Arctii for Soothing Muscles
(Niubang jieji tang)

Ingredients

Fructus Arctii	12 g
Fructus Forsythiae	12 g
Radix Scrophulariae	12 g
Fructus Gardeniae	10 g
Cortex Moutan Radicis	10 g
Spica Prunellae	10 g
Herba Dendrobii	10 g
Herba Schizonepetae	6 g
Herba Menthae	3 g

Decoct the above ingredients in a right amount of water for oral administration.

Efficacy

Clearing away heat and toxic material, expelling wind from the body surface and reducing swelling; mainly for skin infection of the head and neck, accompanied with fever, chilliness, headache, dry mouth, oliguria with reddish urine, red tongue with yellow fur, smooth and rapid pulse, which are attributive to the attack of wind, fire, toxic material and heat.

Indications

1. Applicable to cases of common cold attributive to attack of exogenous wind-heat, which manifest as fever, chilliness, headache, sore-throat, thirst, thinyellow fur on the tongue, floating and rapid pulse.

2. For cases of measles with interrupted eruption, fever, chilliness, sneezing, cough, congestion of conjunctiva, lacrimation, thirst, red tongue with thin yellow fur, floating and rapid pulse, which are attributive to attack of heat and toxic material to the lung and stomach, and retention of the pathogens in the superficies.

3. Also to cases of hordeolum accompanied with fever, chilliness, headache, thirst, red tongue and rapid pulse, which are attributive to attack of heat and toxic material to the eyes.

4. For cases of upper respiratory viral infection and inffluenza attributive to the attack of exogenous wind-heat; and for cases of chalazion and tarsitis attributive to the attack of heat evil and toxic material attack to the eyes.

Interpretation

Arctii acts as the principal drug of the prescription, which can expel wind and heat, eliminate toxic material and relieve swelling. *Schizonepetae*, *Menthae* help *Arctii* to disperse wind-heat from the head and face. *Forsythiae*, *Prunellae*, *Moutan Radicis*, *Gardeniae* and *Scrophulariae*, when used together with *Schizonepetae* and *Menthae*, serve to eliminate heat and toxic material from the head and face, to expel wind from the body surface and to relieve swelling. Because the retention of heat and toxic material can damage the yin-fluid, *Dendrobii* is applied to nourish yin and promote the production of body fluid. When the body fluid is sufficient, the high body temperature may become normal.

Decoction of Coptidis for Detoxification
(Neishu huanglian tang)

Ingredients

Rhizoma Coptidis	9 g
Radix Scutellariae	9 g
Fructus Gardeniae	9 g
Fructus Forsythiae	9 g
Radix Angelicae Sinensis	9 g
Radix Paeoniae Alba	9 g
Radix Aucklandiae	6 g
Herba Menthae	3 g
Radix Platycodi	3 g
Radix Glycyrrhizae	3 g
Radix et Rhizoma Rhei	6 g

Decoct the above ingredients in a right amount of water for oral administration.

Efficacy

Clearing away heat and toxic material, activating blood circulation, relieving swelling and promoting bowel movement.

Indications

To cases of jaundice manifested by bright yellow coloration over the body, fever, thirst, oliguria, reddish urine, constipation, yellow and greasy fur on the tongue, wiry and rapid pulse, which are attributive to the accumulation of dampness - heat.

To cases of appendicitis, liver abscess and lung abscess, to cases of cellulitis, lymphadenitis and mastitis and to cases of acute cholecystitis, icterus infectious hepatitis and cholelithiasis with jaundice attributive to the attack of dampness - heat.

Interpretation

Coptidis, *Scutellariae* and *Gardeniae* have the effects of clearing away heat evil and toxic material from the interior. *Menthae*, *Forsythiae* and *Platycodi* enhance the effects of the above drugs. *Angelicae Sinensis*, *Paeoniae Alba* and *Aucklandiae* serve to promote the circulation of vital qi and blood, and relieve swelling and pain. *Arecae* and *Rhei* promote the circulation of vital qi and bowel movement to purge the fire from below. *Glycyrrhizae* serves to increase the effect of *Rhei*. In sum, this prescription is designed for eliminating heat and toxic material both from the interior and the superficies.

Decoction of Cinnamomi Adding Cinnamomi
(Guizhi jia gui tang)

Ingredients

Ramulus Cinnamomi	15 g
Radix Paeoniae Alba	10 g
Rhizoma Zingiberis Recens	10 g
Radix Glycyrrhizae Praeparata	6 g
Fructus Ziziphi Jujubae	8 pcs

Decoct the above ingredients in a right amount of water for oral administration.

Efficacy

Activating yang - energy, eliminating cold, lowering adverse rising qi; mainly for cases attributive to attack of exogenous cold and adverse rising of cold originally retained in the lower jiao, which manifest feeling of an air flow moving from the lower abdomen upward to the chest and throat, abdominal pain, vomiting, intolerance of cold, white and greasy fur on the tongue, wiry and tense pulse.

Indications

Applicable to cases attributive to accumulation of yin – cold in the collaterals of jueyin, which manifest induration, swelling and pain of the scrotum, preference for warmth and aversion to cold, cold feet, white and greasy fur on the tongue, sunken and wiry pulse.

For cases with palpitation, frightening, feeling of fullness over the chest, cold limbs, white and greasy fur on the tongue, which are attributive to hypofunction of heart – yang, increase the dosage of *Glycyrrhizae Praeparata*.

Also applicable to cases of spasmodic colon and gastro – intestinal neurosis attributive to adverse rising of interior cold accompanied with the attack of exogenous cold; to cases of indirect inguinal hernia and inguinal hernia attributive to the accumulation of yin – cold; and also to cases of sinus arrhythmia and atrioventricular block attributive to hypofunction of heart – yang.

Interpretation

This prescription is composed by adding an extra dose of *Ramulus Cinnamomi* or *Cortex Cinnamomi* to the *Decoction of Ramulus Cinnamomi*. *Ramulus Cinnamomi* is used to disperse cold from the superficies and to lower the adverse rising qi, and serves as the principal drug of the prescription for both symptomatic and causative treatment. *Paeoniae Alba* serves to regulate ying and wei and to promote diaphoresis when it is used together with *Ramulus Cinnamomi*. It can also relieve pain and prevent abnormal rising of liver – qi when it is used together with *Glycyrrhizae Praeparata*. *Zingiberis Recens* can clear away cold, promote sweating and lower the adverse rising qi when it combines with *Ramulus Cinnamomi*, and can regulate ying and wei and warm the spleen and stomach when it combines with *Ziziphi Jujubae*. *Glycyrrhizae Praeparata* used with *Ramulus Cinnamomi* can relieve abnormal throbbing.

Chapter Twenty-one

Decoction for General Antiphlogistic
(Puji xiaodu yin)

Ingredients

Radix Scutellariae	15 g
Rhizoma Coptidis	15 g
Fructus Forsythiae	10 g
Radix Isatidis	10 g
Radix Scrophulariae	10 g
Fructus Arctii	10 g
Exocarpium Citri Grandis	6 g
Radix Glycyrrhizae	6 g
Radix Bupleuri	6 g
Radix Platycodi	6 g
Lasiosphaera seu Calvatia	3 g
Herba Menthae	3 g
Bombyx Batryticatus	3 g
Rhizoma Cimicifugae	3 g

Decoct the above ingredients in a right amount of water for oral administration.

Efficacy

Clearing away heat evil and toxic material, expelling wind evil from the body surface, relieving swelling; mainly for some epidemic diseases attributive to the accumulation of wind, heat and pestilent evil in the head and face, manifested by swelling, redness and pain over the face, chilliness, fever, sore-throat, reddish tongue with white and yellow fur, floating and rapid, strong pulse, etc..

Indications

1. This is a representative prescription for treating the epidemic diseases characterized by swelling and redness of face. When the superficies-syndrome

has subsided and heat-syndrome becomes prominent. *Menthae* and *Bupleuri* should be subtracted and *Flos Lonicerae* added.

2. Applicable to furunculosis of the face and head attributive to upward attack of heat evil and toxic material (usually add *Lonicerae* and *Herba Schizonepetae*, and subtract *Lasiosphaera seu Calvatia* and *Bupleuri*).

3. Also applicable to cases of acute tonsillitis, acute otitis media, acute lymphadentis, mumps, etc., attributive to accumulation of wind-heat and pestilent evil in the head. In cases of mumps complicated by orchitis, add *Fructus Meliae Toosendan* to purge the sthenic fire of liver meridian.

Interpretation

Scutellariae and *Coptidis* are used in large dose to clear away heat evil and toxic material from the upper jiao. *Forsythiae*, *Arctii*, *Bombyx Batryticatus* and *Menthae* serve to expel wind-heat evil from the upper jiao. *Scrophulariae* and *Isatidis* enhance the effects of *Scutellariae*, and *Coptidis*, *Lasiosphaera seu Calvatia*, *Platycodi* and *Glycyrrhizae* are assisted by *Arctii* and *Menthae* to ease the throat. *Exocarpium Citri Grandis* has the effects of regulating vital energy and helps above drugs to expel wind evil and relieve swelling. *Cimicifugae* and *Bupleuri* can expel wind-heat evil and helps the above drugs distributing to the head and face. This is a well-known prescription for clearing away heat evil and toxic material.

Decoction for Purging Liver-fire and Eliminating Dampness (Qing gan sheng shi tang)

Ingredients

Radix Scutellariae	10 g
Fructus Gardeniae	10 g
Radix Angelicae Sinensis	10 g
Radix Paeoniae Alba	10 g
Radix Trichosanthis	10 g

Radix Rehmanniae	20 g
Rhizoma Ligustici Chuanxiong	6 g
Radix Bupleuri	6 g
Radix Gentianae	6 g
Rhizoma Alismatis	6 g
Caulis Akebiae	6 g
Medulla Junci	3 g
Radix Glycyrrhizae	3 g

Decoct the above ingredients in a right amount of water for oral administration.

Efficacy

Clearing away heat and dampness, dispersing the stagnated liver-qi, alleviating pain, activating the circulation of blood and relieving swelling; mainly for cases of scrotitis with chilliness, fever, oliguria, red tongue with yellow and greasy fur, wiry and rapid pulse, which are attributive to downward attack of dampness-heat from the liver meridian and the stagnation of blood and toxic materials.

Indications

1. For cases with induration, pain and swelling of testis, erythema and hotness of the scrotum, accompanied with chilliness, fever, headache, thirst, oliguria with deep-colored urine, red tongue with yellow and greasy fur, wiry and rapid pulse, which are attributive to downward attack of dampness-heat to the collateral of "jueyin" and the stagnation of blood and toxic material, add *Fructus Meliae Toosendan*, or *Semen Citri Grandis*, and omit *Glycyrrhizae* and *Junci*.

2. Also applicable to cases of hydrocele of tunica vaginalis, varicocele of spermatic cord, orchitis, tuberculosis of testis, etc. attributive to downward attack of dampness-heat and stagnation of blood and toxic material.

Interpretation

This prescription is formed by adding *Ligustici Chuanxiong*, *Paeoniae Alba*, *Trichosanthis* and *Junci*, and omitting *Semen Plantaginis* from the *Decoction of Gentianae for purging liver – fire*. In this prescription, *Gardeniae*, *Scutellariae* and *Gentianae* serve to purge the heat – toxic material from the liver meridian, and *Akebiae*, *Junci* and *Alismatis* to eliminate the dampness – toxic material from the lower – jiao. *Angelicae Sinensis*, *Rehmanniae*, *Paeoniae Alba*, *Ligustici Chuanxiong* are used together with *Bupleuri* to activate blood circulation, relieve swelling, disperse the stagnated liver – qi and alleviate pain. *Trichosanthis* has the effects of clearing away heat and eliminating phlegm, and promotes the subsidence of swelling. *Glycyrrhizae* serves to clear away heat and toxic material.

Golden Lock Bolus for Keep Kidney Essence
(Jinsuo gu jing wan)

Ingredients

Semen Astragali Complanati	30 g
Semen Euryales	30 g
Semen Nelumbinis	30 g
Stamen Nelumbinis	15 g
Os Draconis	20 g
Concha Ostreae	20 g

Efficacy

Strengthening kidney essence and stopping nocturnal emission; mainly for cases with hypofunction of kidney, characterized by nocturnal emission, fatigue, sorenss of limbs, lumbago, tinnitus, pale tongue with whitish fur, small and weak pulse.

Indications

1. Applicable to deficiency of both kidney-yin and yang. For cases with deficiency of kidney-yin predominantly, add Fructus Ligustri Lucidi and Fructus Rosae Laevigatae, while for those with deficiency of kidney-yang predominantly, add Fructus Psoraleae and Pulvis of Cornu Cervi. It is not suitabld for nocturnal emission due to hyperactivity of "prime-minister" fire.

2. For cases of leukorrhagia with thin discharge, attributive to deficiency of spleen-yang and yin, omit Stamen Nelumbinis and add Poria and Rhizoma Atractylodis Macrocephalae (in large dosage) to invigorate the spleen and kidney).

3. Applicable to cases of neurasthenia with nocturnal emission, and cervicitis with leukorrhagia, which are attributive to hypofunction of kidney.

Interpretation

Complanati has the effects of invigorating kidney, supporting kidney essence and stopping nocturnal emission. *Semen Nelumbinis* and *Semen Euryales* serve to clear away heart-fire, benefit the kidney and keep heart-fire and kidney-water in balance. *Os Draconis*, *Concha Ostreae* and *Stamen Nelumbinis* can relieve nocturnal emission and calm the mental state. All the above drugs constituent a prescription effective for arresting nocturnal emission.

Zaizao Powder
(Zaizao san)

Ingredients

Radix Astragali seu Hedysari	12 g
Radix codonopsis Pilosulae	10 g
Ramulus Cinnamomi	6 g
Radix Paeoniae Alba	6 g
Radix Aconiti Praeparata	6 g
Rhizoma seu Radix Notopterygii	6 g

Radix Ledebouriellae	6 g
Rhizoma Ligustici Chuanxiong	6 g
Herba Asari	3 g
Radix Glycyrrhizae Praeparata	3 g
Rhizoma Zingiberis Recens	5 pcs
Fructus Ziziphi Jujubae	2 pcs0

Efficacy

Supporting yang – qi to promote sweating, benefiting vital qi and expelling superficial evils from body surface; mainly for cases of common cold of wind – cold type with a yang – deficiency constitution, manifested by fever with predominant chilliness, headache, rigidity of neck, anhidrosis, cold limbs, tiredness, pale complexion, low voice, pale tongue with whitish fur, sunken and weak pulse or floating and large, weak pulse, etc..

Indications

1. Applicable to the early stage of pyogenic infection of skin, manifested by local swelling and pain but no erythema nor heat, with predominant fever, chilliness, anhidrosis, cold limbs, no thirst, thin and whitish fur on the tongue, floating and large, weak pulse, which are attributive to attack of exogenous wind – cold and deficiency of yang – qi in the body.

2. Also indicated for cases of arthralgia with wandering pain, chilliness, fever, anhidrosis, cold limbs, tiredness, flat taste of the mouth, floating and large, weak pulse, which are attributive to attack of wind – cold – dampness evil to a person with yang – deficiency constitution.

3. Also applicable to cases of upper respiratory infection, mumps, rheumatic fever, rheumatoid arthritis, carbuncle, furuncle, acute cellulitis, etc., marked by chilliness and fever, which are attributive to deficiency of yang – qi and the attack of exogenous wind – cold – dampness or wind – cold evil.

Interpretation

This prescription is characterized by simultaneous application of cold – expelling and yang – supporting drugs. *Ramulus cinnamomi*, *Notopterygii*, *Ledebouriellae*, *Asari*, *Ligustici Chuanxiong* and *Zingiberis Recens* are diaphoretics for expelling cold. If only diaphoretics are used for those cases with a yang – deficiency constitution, not only perspiration does not occur but also the deficiency of yang would be aggravated, or even yang exhaustion after profuse sweating may ensue. So *Astragali seu Hedysari* and *Codonopsis* are applied to benefit yang – qi, and *Aconiti* is helpful for strengthen yang and promoting sweating. *Paeoniae Alba* and *Ziziphi Jujubae* can nourish blood. When used together with *Astragali seu Hedysari*, *Paeoniae Alba* exerts an astringent effect to prevent over sweating.

Powder for Antiphlogosis
(Baidu san)

Ingredients

Rhizoma seu Radix Notopterygii	12 g
Radix Angelicae Pubescentis	12 g
Radix Bupleuri	10 g
Radix Peucedani	10 g
Rhizoma Ligustici Chuanxiong	10 g
Radix Codonopsis Pilosulae	6 g
Fructus Aurantii	6 g
Poria	6 g
Radix Platycodi	6 g
Radix Glycyrrhizae	3 g
Herba Menthae	3 g
Rhizoma Zingiberis Recens	3 pcs

Decoct the above ingredients in a right amount of water for oral administration.

Efficacy

Benefiting vital qi and expelling the evils from the body surface, eliminating the wind and dampness evil; mainly for cases with insufficiency of healthy qi and attacked by exogenous wind, cold and dampness evil, which are manifested by chilliness, fever, headache, no sweating, general aching, stuffy nose, heavy voice, productive cough, whitish and greasy fur on the tongue, floating and weak pulse, etc..

Indications

1. Applicable to skin infections which are attributive to wind – cold – dampness superficies – syndrome.
2. By adding *Fructus Forsythiae* and *Flos Lonicerae*, and omitting *Codonopsis Pilosulae*, another prescription named *Powder of Forsythiae for Antiphlogosis* is formed. It is indicated for the initial stage of skin infections attributive to virulent heat evil attacking the superficies.
3. By adding *Herba Schizonepetae* and *Radix Ledebouriellae* and omitting *Codonopsis Pilosulae*, *Zingiberis Recens* and *Menthae*, another prescription named *Powder of Schizonepetae and Ledebouriellae for Antiphlogosis* is formed. It is indicated for affections of exogenous wind, cold and dampness evil, which are manifested by chilliness, fever, heavy sensation of head and body, cough, heavy voice, white and greasy fur on the tongue, wiry and tense pulse, etc..
4. Also applicable to cases of influenza, emphysema complicated by infection, malaria, acute cellulitis, etc., which are attirbutive to the affection of wind, cold and dampness evil in cases of the insufficiency of healthy qi.

Interpretation

Notopterygii and *Angelicae Pubescentis* not only can disperse wind – cold evil, but also can eliminate dampness and relieve pain. The former distributes upwardly and the latter downwardly, and they act on the whole body when used together. A small amount of *Codonopsis Pilosulae* is applied together with *Bupleuri*, *Ligustici Chuanxiong*, *Zingiberis Recens* and *Menthae* to invigorate vital qi and expel the evil factors from the body surface by sweating. A small amount of *Poria* is applied together with those drugs of *Peucedani*, *Aurantii* and *Platycodi* to eliminate sputum and relieve cough. *Radix Glycyrrhizae* serves to regulate the other drugs. This prescription combines both tonics and diaphoretics together, and possesses the advantage of producing sweating but not damaging the healthy qi, and that of supporting the healthy qi but not retaining the evils.

Pill of Six Miraculous Drugs
(Liushen wan)

Ingredients

Margarita	4.5 g
Calculus Bovis	4.5 g
Moschus	4.5 g
Realgar	3 g
Borneolum Syntheticum	3 g
Venenum Bufonis	3 g

Coated with burnt herbal powder.

Efficacy

Clearing away heat and toxic material, relieving swelling and alleviating pain; mainly for cases of scarlet fever and tonsillitis with red tongue and rapid pulse, which are attributive to the accumulation of phlegm, fire and toxic material.

Indications

1. The prescription cannot be applied as a decoction for oral use. Some ingredients such as *Realgar* and *Venenum Bufonis* are poisonous, so it should not be taken in alrge dose nor for a long period and is contraindicated for pregnant women.

2. Applicable to carbuncle, furuncle, abscess of breast, and various local infection of unknown origin, which are attributive to accumulation of phlegm, fire and toxic material.

3. Also applicable to cases of pharyngitis, follicular stomatitis, mastitis, nasopharyngeal carcinoma, lung cancer, etc. which are attributive to accumulation of phlegm, fire and toxic material.

The recipe can be modified to deal with influenza, epidemic encephalitis B epidemic cerebrospinal meningitis, pneumonia and septicemia indicating excessive heat syndrome in the qi system, and also with the treatment of stomatitis, periodontitis, gastritis, diabetes and others which pertain to stomach heat syndrome.

Interpretation

Calculus Bovis, *Realgar* and *Venenum Bufonis* are principal drugs in the prescrription, which have strong and fast effect of eliminating toxic materials and dispersing the accumulation of evils. *Calculus Bovis* can eliminate heat – phlegm, *Realgar* can disperse the stagnated substance, and *Venenum Bufonis* can relieve swelling and alleviate pain. They all are potent agents for clearing away heat and dispelling toxic material, and serve as the principal drugs of the prescription. *Margarita* can clear away heart – fire and eliminate phlegm when it combines with *Calculus Bovis*. *Borneolum Syntheticum* can disperse heat and alleviate pain, and also increase the effect of the other drugs with it combining with *Moschus*. *Burnt herbal powder* has the effect of dispersing the stagnated substance and easing the throat, and is especially good for the infection of oral cavity. In sum, the prescription has a strong detoxifying and swelling – subsiding effect by utilizing the fragrant nature of the ingredients.

Cautions

It is not advisable for those whose exterior syndrome is not relieved, nor for those who have fever due to blood – deficiency or cold syndrome with pseudo – heat symptoms.

Decoction of Phragmitis
(Weijing tang)

Ingredients

Rhizoma Phragmitis	60 g
Semen Coicis	30 g
Semen Benincasae	30 g
Semen Persicae	10 g

Decoct the above ingredients in a right amount of water for oral administration.

Efficacy

Clearing away lung-heat and eliminating sputum, removing blood stasis and pus; mainly for cases of pulmonary abscess with expectoration of foul, purulent and bloody sputum, chest pain aggravated by coughing, red tongue with yellow, greasy fur, smooth and rapid pulse.

Indications

1. This is a typical prescription for pulmonary abscess. For cases without formation of pus, add *Radix Platycodi* and *Bulbus Fritillariae Cirrhosae* to enhance the effect of eliminating the sputum and the pus.

2. For cases of measles after the occurrence of skin eruptions, but still with fever, productive cough, red tongue with yellow greasy fur, smooth and rapid pulse, which are attributive to lung-heat, omit *Persicae* and add *Cortex Mori Radicis* and *Bulbus Fritillariae Thunbergii*.

3. Also applicable to cases of lobar pneumonia, bronchitis, whooping cough, etc. which are attributive to lung-heat.

Interpretation

Phragmitis has the effects of clearing away lung-heat and is the principal remedy for pulmonary abscess. *Benincasae* eliminates sputum and pus. *Coicis* clears away heat-evil and promotes diuresis. *Persciae* removes blood stasis and pus. All of these three seeds can also move the bowels and eliminate the pus and blood stasis through defecation. These constitute and ideal prescription for pulmonary abscess of sputum-heat pattern or sputum-blood-stasis pattern. The abscess can be dispersed when the pus is not yet formed, and the pus can be eliminated when the abscess is formed.

Powder of Lonicerae and Forsythiae
(Yinqiao san)

Ingredients

Flos Lonicerae	12 g
Fructus Forsythiae	12 g
Fructus Arctii	10 g
Semen Sojae Praeparatum	10 g
Rhizoma Phragmitis	10 g
Radix Platycodi	5 g
Herba Menthae	5 g
Herba Lophatheri	5 g
Radix Glycyrrhizae	5 g
Spica Schizonepetae	5 g

Efficacy

Expelling wind and heat evil, clearing away heat evil and toxic material; mainly for cases due to exogenous wind and heat evil, which are manifested by fever, mild chilliness, sore-throat, headache, thirst, red tip of the tongue with thin white fur or thin yellowish fur, floating and rapid pulse, etc..

Indications

1. The therapeutic principle of this prescription is reasonable, the concept of compatibility is strict and its curative effect is fruitful, and has become a typical recipe for common cold of wind-heat type. For cases with extreme thirst, add *Radix Trichosanthis* to promote the production of saliva and quench thirst; for cases with sore-throat, add *Radix Scrophulariae* to clear away the heat evil and ease the throat.

2. For the initial stage of measles attributive to stagnation of wind and heat evil in the superficies, which is manifested by fever, thirst and incomplete eruption, add *Radix Puerariae* to let out the eruptions.

3. For cases at the onset of skin infections attributive to super ficies-syndrome of wind-heat type, add *Herba Taraxaci* or *Folium Isatidis* to clear away heat evil and toxic material, and dispersing the accumulation of evils.

4. Also applicable to cases of acute tonsillitis, influenza, mumps, measles, encephalitis B epidemic meningitis and acute suppurative infection, which are attributive to wind-heat syndrome of the superficies.

Interpretation

Lonicerae and *Forsythiae* are selected as principal drugs which have mild action to let the evil out of the body and clear away heat evil and toxic material, so as to prevent the evil from attacking the interior. *Schizonepetae*, *Menthae* and *Sojae Praeparatum* can expel the evils from the surface of the body owing to their acrid flavour. *Arctii*, *Platycodi* and *Glycyrrhizae* have the effects of clearing away heat evil and toxic material to ease the throat. *Lophatheri* and *Phragmitis* have the effects of clearing away heat evil and promoting the production of body fluid to relieve thirst. This prescription constitutes an acrid-cool remedy by combining the drugs of clearing away heat evil and toxic material with those of expelling the evil from the body surface. This model of compatibility exerts a great influence upon the later generation, and many new set prescriptions for common cold are composed of its modifications.

Powder of Ledebouriellae for Dispersing the Superficies
(Fangfeng tongsheng san)

Ingredients

Radix Ledebouriellae	10 g
Fructus Forsythiae	10 g
Fructus Gardeniae	10 g
Herba Schizonepetae	6 g
Herba Ephedrae	6 g
Rhizoma Ligustici Chuanxiong	6 g
Radix Angelicae Sinensis	6 g
Radix Paeoniae Alba	6 g
Rhizoma Atractylodis Macrocephalae	6 g
Radix et Rhizoma Rhei	6 g
Natrii Sulfas	6 g
Radix Scutellariae	6 g
Talcum	20 g
Gypsum Fibrosum	15 g
Herba Menthae	3 g
Radix Platycodi	3 g
Radix Glycyrrhizae	3 g
Rhizoma Zingiberis Recens	3 pcs

Decoct the above ingredients in a right amount of water for oral administration.

Efficacy

Expelling wind from the body surface, clearing away heat and promoting bowel movement; mainly for sthenia – syndrome of both the superficies and the interior after the attack of exogenous wind – heat and the retention of heat in the interior, which is manifested by aversion to cold, fever, dizziness, bitter and dry mouth, conjunctivitis, sore – throat, feeling of oppression over the chest, constipation, dysuria with reddish urine, red tongue with white or yellow fur, floating and smooth, rapid pulse.

Indications

1. Applicable to cases of early stage of superficial pyogenic infection with local signs of inflammation, chilliness, fever, bitter mouth, constipation, oliguria, red tongue with white fur, floating and rapid pulse.

2. Also indicated for cases of urticaria and eczema with thin and white fur on the tongue, floating and rapid pulse, which are attributive to simultaneous existence of sthenia - syndrome in the superficies and the interior.

3. Also applicable to cases of influenza, poliomyelitis, infectious mononucleosis, mumps, acute cellulitis, erysipelas, acute lymphangitis, etc., which are attributive to simultaneous existence of sthenia - syndrome in the superficies and the interior after attack of exogenous wind - heat and retention of heat in the body.

Interpretation

Ledebouriellae, *Schizonepetae*, *Ephedrae*, *Zingiberis Recens* and *Menthae* serve to expel wind by sweating. *Rhei* and *Natrii Sulfas* eliminate the internal heat by purgation, and *Gardeniae* and *Talcum* clear away heat by diuresis. *Platycodi*, *Gypsum Fibrosum*, *Scutellariae* and *Forsythiae* can clear away heat from the lung and stomach. All the above drugs act together to eliminate heat from the upper and the lower part of the body, and treat both the superficies and the interior syndrome. *Angelicae Sinensis*, *Ligustici Chuanxiong* and *Paeoniae Alba* have the effects of expelling wind and nourishing blood, and *Atractylodis Macrocephalae* and *Glycyrrhizae* serve to strengthen the spleen and regulating the stomach; they cooperate each other to exert a diaphoretic effect without damaging the superficies, and exert a purgative effect without impairing the interior. In sum, this prescription involves the therapeutic principles of diaphoretic, heat - eliminating, purgative and tonifying simultaneously, aiming at clearing away the internal heat chiefly. The application of *Natrii Sulfas* and *Rhei* is for purging heat.

White Tiger Decoction
(Baihu tang)

Ingredients

Gypsum Fibrosum	30 g
Rhizoma Anemarrhenae	9 g
Radix Glycyrrhizae Praeparata	3 g
Semen Oryzae Nonglutionosae	9 g

All the above drugs are to be decocted in water for oral administration.

Efficacy

Clearing away heat and promoting the production of body fluid.

Indications

Yangming channel diseases marked by high fever, flushed face, polydipsia, profuse perspiration, aversion to heat and full forceful pulse. It can be modified to treat influenza, epidemic encephalitis B, epidemic cerebrospinal meningitis, pneumonia and septicemia indicating excessive heat syndrome in the qi system.

Cautions

It is not advisable for those whose exterior syndrome is not relieved, nor for those who have fever due to blood - deficiency or cold syndrome with pseudo - heat symptoms.

Decoction of Gypsum Fibrosum and Three Yellows
(Sanhuang shigao tang)

Ingredients

Gypsum Fibrosum (decocted first	30 g
Radix Scutellariae	10 g
Rhizoma Coptidis	10 g
Cortex Phellodendri	10 g
Fructus Gardeniae	10 g
Semen Sojae Praeparatum	10 g
Herba Ephedrae	3 g
Rhizoma Zingiberis Recens	3 pcs
Fructus Ziziphi Jujubae	2 pcs
Folium Camelliae Sinensis	6 g

Decoct the above ingredients in a right amount of water for oral administration.

Efficacy

Expelling the pathogens from both the interior and the superficies, purging fire and eliminating toxic materials; mainly for seasonal febrile diseases involving both the interior and superficies, which manifest as high fever, chilliness, anhidrosis, flushed cheeks, dryness of teeth and nose, extreme thirst, severe headache, irritability or even mania, red tongue with yellow fur, bounding and rapid or smooth and rapid pulse.

Indications

1. For cases with yang macules which are punctate or pieces and bright red in colour, accompanied with high fever, thirst, flushed cheeks, conjunctival congestion, red or crimson tongue with yellow fur, bounding and rapid pulse, which are attributive to stagnation of heat in the *yangming* channel involving *yingfen* and *xuefen*, use *Radix Rehmanniae* instead of *Ephedrae* and *Sojae Praepara-*

tum.

2. Also applicable to cases suffering from common cold, encephalitis **B**, typhoid fever and paratyphoid fever with high fever, which are attributive to attack of potent heat to both interior and the superficies; and to cases of epidemic hemorrhagic fever, typhus fever, which are attributive to the stagnation of heat in the *yangming* channel involving *yingfen* and *xuefen*.

3. Applicable to infections of skin and subcutaneous tissues acccompanied with high fever, irritability, extreme thirst, oliguria with reddish urine, red tongue with yellow fur, wiry and rapid pulse, which are attributive to retnetion of heat and toxic material in the superficies when the pathogens are potent and the healthy energy is still strong.

Interpretation

Gypsum Fibrosum can clear away the interior heat and acts as the chief drug of the prescription. *Ephedrae* and *Sojae Praeparatum* are applied to promote sweating and discharge the heat outside. The above three durgs used together can expel heat from both the interior and the superficies. Since there is a large amount of heat in the triple-jiao, *Scutellariae* is applied to clear away the heat in the upper-jiao. *Gardeniae* and *Camelliae Sinensis* can discharge the heat of triple-jiao from the urine. *Zingiberis* and *Ziziphi Jujubae* serve to regulate *ying* and *wei*.

Decoction of Ginseng for Nourishing Qi and Ying
(Renshen yang rong tang)

Ingredients

Radix Paeoniae Alba	15 g
Radix Rehmanniae Praeparata	15 g
Radix Codonopsis Pilosulae	10 g
Radix Astragali seu Hedysari	10 g
Rhizoma Atractylodis Macrocephalae	10 g

Poria	10 g
Radix Angelicae Sinensis	10 g
Exocarpium Citri Grandis	6 g
Fructus Schisandrae	6 g
Radix Glycyrrhizae Praeparata	3 g
Cortex Cinnamomi	3 g
Radix Polygalae	3 g
Rhizoma Zingiberis Recens	3 pcs
Fructus Ziziphi Jujubae	3 pcs

Decoct the above ingredients in a right amount of water for oral administration.

Efficacy

Benefiting qi, tonifying blood, strengthening spleen and nourishing heart; mainly for consumptive diseases manifested by palpitation, amnesia, insomnia, dreaminess, tiredness, profuse sweating, poor appetite, shortness of breath, dyspnea upon exertion, pale tongue, sunken and weak pulse, which are attributive to insufficiency of qi and blood, and hypofunction of heart and spleen.

Indications

Applicable to cases of irregular (or delayed) menstruation with scanty pale discharge, sallow complexion, palpitation, dizziness, shortness of breath, fatigue, poor appetite, pale tongue, which are attributive to deficiency of liver - blood and spleen - qi and failure of releasing stagnated qi and controlling blood.

2. Also indicated for the late stage of pyogenic infection of skin when the acute inlammation subsides but the qi and blood are deficient, which manifest lesion with discharge of thin purulent fluid, dark greyish coloration but without granulation, and accompanied with lusterless complexion and pale tongue.

3. Also applicable to cases of pulmonary tuberculosis, rheumatic heart diseases, gastric ulcer, tuberculous abscess, carbuncle, phlebeurysma of the lower limbs, etc. which are attributive to deficiency of qi and blood.

Interpretation

The prescription is composed by omitting *Rhizoma Ligustici Chuanxiong* and adding *Astragali seu Hedysari*, *Cortex Cinnamomi*, *Citri Grandis*, *Schisandrae* and *Polygalae* to the *Decoction of Eight Ingredients for Tonifying Qi and Blood*. *Ligustici Chuanxiong* is omitted because the effect of activating blood circulation is not desired. The effect of tonifying blood and promoting blood production is obtained when *Astragali seu Hedysari* is used together with *Angelicae Sinensis*. *Cortex Cinnamomi* used together with *Zingiberis Recens*, *Ziziphi Jujubae* can accelerate the growth of qi and blood. *Polygalae* and *Schisandrae* adding to *Codonopsis Pilosulae* and *Astragali seu Hedysari* serve to benefit the heart – qi and tranquilizing. *Citri Grandis* is used for regulating qi and stomach to decrease the indigestibility of the tonics.

Ease Powder
(Xiao Yao San)

Ingredients

Radix bupleuri	15 g
Radix Angelicae Sinensis	15 g
Radix Paeoniae Alba	15 g
Poria	15 g
Rhizoma Atractylodis Macrocephalae	15 g
Rhizoma Zingiberis Recens Praeparata	3 g
Herba Menthae	3 g
Radix Glycyrrhizae Praeparata	6 g

Grind the above drugs except *ginger* and *peppermint* into powder take 6 to 9 grams each time with a decoction in small amount of roasted *ginger* and *peppermint*.

Efficacy

Soothing the liver disperse depressed qi, and invigorating the spleen to nourish the blood.

Indications

Stagnation of the liver - qi with deficiency of the blood marked by hypochondriac pain, headache, dizziness, bitter mouth, dry throat, mental weariness and poor appetite, or alternate attacks of chills and fever, or irregular menstruation, distension in the breast, light redness of the tongue, taut and feeble pulse.

Patients with chronic hepatitis, Pleuritis, chronic gastritis, neurosis, irregular menstruation marked by symptoms of stagnation of liver - qi with deficiency of the blood can be treated by the modified recipe.

Interpretation

Bupleurum root in the recipe soothes the liver to disperse the depressed qi. *Chinese yam* and *White peony root* nourish the blood and the liver. The joint use of the three drugs is able to treat the primary cause of stagnation of the liver - qi and deficiency of the blood. *Poria* and *Bighead atractylodes rhizome* strengthen the middle - jiao and reinforce the spleen so as to enrich the source of growth and development of the qi and blood. *Roasted ginger* regulates the stomach and warms the middle - jiao. *Peppermint* assists *Bupleurum root* in soothing the liver to disperse the depressed qi. *Prepared licorice root* can not only assist *Bighead atractylodes rhizome* and *Poria* in replenishing qi and invigorating the middle - warmer but also coordinate the effects of all the drugs in the recipe.

Modern researches have proved that the recipe has remarkable effects of nourishing the liver, tranquilizing the mind and relieving spasm. It is also effective in promoting digestion, coordinating uterine function, nourishing blood, strengthening the stomach and so on.

Decoction of Aneglicae Pubescentis and Taxilli
(Duhuo Jisheng Tang)

Ingredients

Radix Angelicae Pubescentis	10 g
Cortex Eucommiae	10 g
Radix Achyranthis Bidentatae	10 g
Radix Gentianae Macrophyllae	10 g
Poria	10 g
Radix Ledebouriellae	10 g
Radix Angelicae Sinensis	10 g
Radix Codonopsis Pilosulae	10 g
Radix Paeoniae Alba	10 g
Ramulus Taxilli	18 g
Radix Rehmanniae	18 g
Lignum Cinnamomi	1.5 g
Rhizoma Ligustici Chuanxiong	6 g
Herba Asari	3 g
Radix Glycyrrhizae	3 g

Decoct the above ingredients in a right amount of water for oral administration.

Efficacy

Expelling wind – dampness evil, relieving arthralgia, benefiting the liver and kidney, invigorating vital energy and blood; mainly for prolonged arthralgia of wind – cold – dampness type with hypofunction of liver and kidney and insufficiency of vital energy and blood, which is manifested as cold pain over the loin and joints, limited mobility and flaccidity of joints, or numbness, aversion to cold and desire for warmth, pale tongue with whitish fur, small and weak pulse.

Indications

1. Applicable to cases of stroke manifested by hemiplegia, numbness, spasm of limbs, pale tongue with whitish fur, small and weak pulse, which are attributive to deficiency of both the liver and the kidney, and attack of wind evil to the meridians.

2. Also applicable to cases of chronic rheumatic arthritis, rheumatic sciatica, lumbar strain, prolapse of lumbar intervertebral disc, etc., marked by cold pain over the loin and knees, which are attributive to prolonged bi - syndrome with deficiency of both the liver and the kidney and insufficiency of vital energy and blood.

Interpretation

Angelicae Pubescentis, *Ledebouriellae* and *Gentianae Macrophyllae* have the effects of expelling wind and dampness, *Asari* expels wind - cold evil from the yin - channel and eliminates wind - dampness evil from the muscles and tendons; the above three drugs used together exert an analgesic effect for rheumatism of wind - cold - dampness type evil and relieving pain. Prolonged rheumatism (attack of wind - cold - dampness evil) may aggravate the deficiency of liver and kidney, so *Ramulus Taxilli*, *Achyranthis Bidentatae* and *Eucommiae* are applied to tonify the liver and kidney, strengthen the tendons and bones, *Codonopsis Pilosulae*, *Poria*, *Glycyrrhizae* to invigorate healthy energy, and *Rehmanniae*, *Angelicae Sinensis* and *Paeoniae Alba* to nourish blood and activate blood circulation. Moreover, *Ligustici Chuanxiong* and *Lignum Cinnamomi* are added to warm and dredge the vessels and expel wind evil. In sum, the prescription serves as both symptomatic and causative therapy for arthralgia by supplementing vital energy and blood, invigorating liver and kidney, and eliminating wind.

Decoction for Pus Drainage and Relieving Pain
(Tuoli ding tong tang)

Ingredients

Radix Rehmanniae Praeparata	18 g
Radix Angelicae Sinensis	12 g
Radix Paeoniae Alba	12 g
Rhizoma Ligustici Chuanxiong	8 g
Pericarpium Papaveris	8 g
Cortex Cinnamomi	3 g
Olibanum	3 g
Myrrhae	3 g

Decoct the above ingredients in a right amount of water for oral administration.

Efficacy

Nourishing blood, promoting granulation, eliminating blood stasis and relieving pain; mainly for unhealed carbuncle after rupture with thin purulent bloody discharge, severe pain, poor granulation, pale tongue, small and rapid pulse.

Indications

1. Applicable to cases of dysmenorrhea with oligomenorrhea and darkish discharge, fatigue, pale or darkish tongue, sunken and small, unsmooth pulse, which are attributive to deficiency and stagnation of blood.

2. Also applicable to cases of thromboangiitis obliterans, chronic ulcer of lower extremity and tuberculosis of cervical lymph nodes with unhealed wound and poor granulation and case of endometriosis, endometritis, hysteromyoma and vegetative neurosis marked by dysmenorrhe, which are attributive to deficiency and stagnation of blood.

Interpretation

Olibanum and *Myrrhae* promote blood circulation and remove blood stasis to relieve pain. *Rehmanniae Praeparata*, *Angelicae Sinensis*, *paeoniae Alba* and *Ligustici Chuanxiong* are used for nourishing blood to promote granulation and help the first two drugs to promote blood circulation and relieve pain. A small dosage of *Cinnamomi* combined with *Rehmannaie Praeparata* and *Angelicae Sinensis* has the effects of activating the blood and vital qi circulation and promoting granulation. *Pericarpium Papaveris* exerts a prompt astringent and analgesic effect.

Xiaojin Pellet
(Xiao jin dan)

Ingredients

Resina Liquidambaris	3 g
Radix Aconiti Kusnezoffii	6 g
Olibanum	6 g
Myrrha	6 g
Faeces Trogropterori	10 g
Radix Angelicae Sinensis	10 g
Lumbricus	10 g
Carbonized Chinese ink	1 g

The above drugs are ground into powder and prepared as pellets, taken with rice wine.

Efficacy

Eliminating cold, expelling phlegm, removing blood stasis and reducing swelling; mainly for multiple abscesses, subcutaneous nodules, scrofula, and osteomyelitis with local pain and swelling, which are attributive to retention of phlegm-dampness evil in the meridians.

Indications

1. Applcable to cases of stomachache with tenderness, or hematemesis with purplish-dark discharge, darkish tongue with white and smooth fur, unsmooth pulse, which are attributive to stagnation of blood and phlegm.

2. Also applicable to cases of cold abscess, tuberculous lymphadenitis, tuberculosis of joints and chronic osteomyelitis attributive to the stagnation of cold-phlegm and dampness; also to cases of gastric cancer and breast carcinoma attribvutive to the stagnation of blood and phlegm.

Interpretation

Aconit Kusnezoffii has the effects of eliminating cold and dampness, dredging the passage of meridians, reducing swelling and alleviating pain. *Momordicae and Resina Liquidambaris* serve to reduce swelling and alleviate pain. *Moschus* can reopen the meridians, remove blood stasis and relieve swelling. The above four drugs serve as the principal drugs in the prescription. *Lumbricus* used together with *Aconiti Kusnezoffii* can eliminate phlegm and cold, dredge the passage of meridians and activate yang. *Carbonized Chinese ink* used together with *Moschus* can eliminate dampness, remove blood stasis and reduce swelling. *Olibanum*, *Myrrha*, *Faeces Trogopterori* and *rice wine* can activate blood circulation, reduce swelling and alleviate pain. *Angelicae Sinensis* is applied for nourishing blod, so that the healthy qi will not be impaired when blood stasis is removed by other drugs. It also enhances the effect of *Aconiti Kusnezoffii*.

Decoction for Warming Yang
(Yang he tang)

Ingredients

Radix Rehmanniae Praeparata	30 g
Cortex Cinnamomi	3 g
Herba Ephedrae	2 g

Colla Cornus Cervi	9 g
Semen Sinapis Albae	6 g
Rhizoma Zingiberis Praeparata	2 g
Radix Glycyrrhizae	3 g

Decoct the above ingredients in a right amount of water for oral administration.

Efficacy

Warming yang, tonifying blood, expelling cold and dispersing stagnation; mainly for yin type carbuncle, bone carbuncle, multiple abscesses and arthroncus of knee joint, attributive to deficiency of blood and stagnation of cold evil, manifested by local and not well-demarcated swelling, no change of color and temperature, no pain or just mild aching, pale tongue with whitish and smooth fur, sunken and slow pulse.

Indications

1. For cases of yin type carbuncle with pale tongue, floating and large pulse, complicated by deficiency of vital qi, add raw **Radix Astragali seu Hedysari** to benefit vital qi and promot pus drainage.

2. Applicable to cases of dyspneic cough with profuse and thin sputum, which are attributive to hypofunction of both lung and kidney with retention of dampness-phlegm, in this case the prescription is used for warming and invigorating the lung and kidney, eliminating sputum and relieving dyspnea. It may also be applied for cases of bi-syndrome and dysmenorrhea attributive to blood deficiency and cold-stagnation, and serves to warm yang, tonify blood, expel cold evil and arrest pain in this case.

3. Also applicable to cases of deep abscess, bone tuberculosis, chronic osteomyelitis, rheumatic arthritis, tuberculosis of knee joint, etc. which are attributive to blood-deficiency and cold-stagnation.

Interpretation

Rehmanniae Praeparata has the effcts of warming and tonifying ying-blood and inhibiting diaphoretic effect of *Ephedrae*, so that the latter preserves the action of warming the striae. *Colla Cornus Cervi* can produce essence substance, nourish bone marrow and blood, and support yang. It also inhibits the "dispersing" effect of *Cinnamomi* and *Zingiberis* and renders them just for warming and dredging the channels, and removing the stagnation of cold and phlegm. In turn, *Cinnamomi* and *Zingiberis* render *Rehmanniae Praeparata* and *Colla Cornus Cervi* exerting tonic effect but not greasy. *Ephedrae* distributes to the superficis, while *Rehmanniae Praeparata* to the interior. Two drugs help each other to warm and dredgethe striae and channels. *Sinapis Albae* serve to eliminate phlegm and disperse the stagnation of evil. *Glycyrrhizae* is used rawly just for detoxification. In summary, this prescription does not stress on the elimination of toxic material for the treatment of yin type carbuncle. It composed of drugs for warming yang, nourishing blood, dispersing cold and dredging stagnation of evil, thus embodies the therapeutic principle that the root cause of the disease must be aimed at.

Decoction of Persicae for Purgation
(Taohe chengqi tang)

Ingredients

Semen Persicae	12 g
Radix et Rhizoma Rhei	12 g
Ramulus Cinnamomi	10 g
Radix Glycyrrhizae Praeparata	6 g
Natrii Sulfas	6 g

Decoct the above ingredients in a right amount of water for oral administration.

Efficacy

Eliminating blood stasis and purging heat evil; mainly for blood-stagnation syndrome due to accumulation of blood stasis and heat evil in the lower jiao, which is manifested by distending pain over the lower abdomen, irritability, sunken and solid pulse.

Indications

1. For cases of preceded menstrual cycle, amenorrhea, metrorrhagia, etc., attributive to combination of blood stasis and heat evil in the lower jiao, omit *Glycyrrhizae* from the prescription and add *Radix Angelicae Sinensis* to regulate meenstruation, activate blood circulation, eliminate blood stasis and stop bleeding.

2. For cases of abdominal pain after operation due to blood stasis, or trauma (especially the early stage of fracture of thoracic or lumbar vertebrae), which are attributive to combination of blood stasis and heat evil, omit *Glycyrrhizae* and add *Radix Cyathulae* to activate blood circulation and eliminate blood stasis, and let the blood flowing downwards.

3. Applicable to cases of hematemesis, headache, congestion of conjunctiva, which are attributive to upward attack of blood stasis and heat evil.

4. Also applicable to cases of intestinal obstruction, pelvic cellulitis, appendicitis, etc. with abdominal pain, or cases of retention of placenta, dysfunctional uterine bleeding, etc. with headache or bleeding from the gum, which are attributive to combination or upward attack of blood stasis and heat evil.

Major Decoction for Purging Down Digestive Qi
(Da chengqi tang)

Ingredients

Radix et Rhizoma Rhei	12 g
Cortex Magnoliae Officinalis	15 g

Fructus Aurantii Immaturus   12 g
Natrii Sulfas   9 g

Decoct the above ingredients in a right amount of water for oral administration.

Efficacy

Expelling pathogenic heat and loosening the bowel, promoting the circulation of qi to purge accumulation in the bowels.

Indications

1. Excessive – heat syndrome of *yangming – fu* organ, manifested by constipation, frequent wind through the anus, feeling of fullness in the abdomen, abdominal pain with tenderness and guarding, tidal fever, delirium, polyhidrosis of hands and feet, prickled tongue with yellow dry fur or dry black tongue coating with fissures, deep and forceful pulse.
2. Syndrome of fecal impaction due to heat with watery discharge, manifested by watery discharge of terribly foul odor accompnaied by abdominal distension and pain with tenderness and guarding, dry mouth and tongue, smooth and forceful pulse.
3. Cold limbs due to excess of heat, convulsion, mania and other symptoms belonging to excess syndrome of interior heat.

Equally, this recipe can be modified to deal with infectious or non – infectious febrile diseasesin their climax marked by accumulation of heat type, and in the treatment of paralytic, simple and obliterative intestinal obstructions.

Interpretation

Rhei has the purgative effect and eliminating heat, but cannot induce an immediate purgation since it only promotes the peristalsis of large intestine and cannot soften the dry feces. While *Natrii Sulfas* can creat a hypertonic condition in the large intestine and retain enough amount of water to softne the dry feces. hence the two drugs used together may give an immediate purgation. Moreover,

Magnoliae Officinalis and *Aurantii Immaturus* have the effects of promoting vital qi circulation and relieving distension in the abdomen, so as to regulate the function of the gastrointestine, and enhance the effect of *Rhei* and *Natrii Sulfas*.

Major Decoction of Bupleurum
(Da chaihu tang)

Ingredients

Radix Bupleuri	15 g
Radix Scutellariae	9 g
Radix Paeoniae Alba	9 g
Rhizoma Pinelliae	9 g
Fructus Aurantii Immaturus Praeparata	9 g
Radix et Rhizoma Rhei	6 g
Rhizoma Zingiberis Recens	15 g
Fructus Ziziphi Jujubae	5 pcs

Decoct the above ingredients in a right amount of water for oral administration.

Efficacy

Treating *shaoyang* disease by mediation and purging away internal stasis of heat.

Indications

Shaoyang and *yangming* diseases complex marked by alternate attacks of chills and fever, fullness and oppression in the chest, hypochondriac discomfort, frequent vomiting, mental depression and dysphoria, epigastric fullness and pain or epigastric rigidity, constipation or diarrhea due to interior cold and exterior heat, yellow tongue fur, stringy and forceful pulse.

Patients with acute cholecystitis, cholelithiasis, acute pancreatitis and infectionof abdominal activity marked by the above-mentioned symptoms can be treated by the modified recipe.

Pill of Stephaniae Tetrandrae, Zanthoxyli, Lepidii seu Descurainiae and Rhei
(Ji jiao li huang wan)

Ingredients

Radix Stephaniae Tetrandrae	10 g
Semen Zanthoxyli	10 g
Semen Lepidii seu Descurainiae	10 g
Radix et Rhizoma Rhei	6 g

Decoct the above ingredients in a right amount of water for oral administration.

Efficacy

Eliminating the retained fluid and discharging the evils from the lower part; mainly for phlegm-retention syndrome manifested by abdominal fullness, loose stools, dry mouth and tongue, sunken and wiry pulse, which is attributive to retention of fluid in the intestines when the healthy energy is still strong and the evil is hyperactive.

Indications

1. Applicable to cases of dyspneic cough accompanied by feeling of fullness over the chest, inability to lie flat, profuse expectoration, constipation, oliguria, yellow and greasy fur, wiry and smooth pulse, which are attributive to retention of fluid in the thorax.

2. Also inidcated for cases of dysuria accompanied withdyspnea, constipation, floating and smooth pulse, which are attributive to stagnation of phlegm-

heat in the lung, and adverse rising of qi.

3. Also applicable to cases of cirrhosis of liver, chronic nephritis, idiopathic edema, tuberculous pleurisy, lung cancer with pleuralmetastasis, acute glomerular nephritis, urinary infection, etc. which are attributive to fluid or phlegm retention.

Powder of Bupleuri for Dispersing the Depressed Liver – Qi
(Chaihu shugan san)

Ingredients

Radix Bupleuri	10 g
Fructus Aurantii	10 g
Rhizoma Ligustici Chuanxiong	10 g
Exocarpium Citri Grandis	10 g
Rhizoma Cyperi	10 g
Radix Paeoniae Alba	15 g
Radix Glycyrrhizae Praeparata	6 g

Decoct the above ingredients in a right amount of water for oral administration.

Efficacy

Dispersing the stagnated liver – qi, regulating vital qi, activating blood circulation and relieving pain; mainly for ceses due to stagantion of liver – qi and vital qi manifested by fullness of breast, hypochondriac pain, or dysmenorrhea, or stomachache, and for cases due to stagnation of liver and gallbladder heat manifested by alternating episodes of chills and fever.

Indications

1. This prescription and *Powder for Treating Yang Exhaustion* both have the similar action and indication, but the former, owning to the action of *Bupleuri*,

ahs a stronger effect on dispersing the stagnated liver – qi, regulating the vital qi and adtivating blood circulation. It is frequently applied for the cases of menoxenia or distending pain of the breast.

2. For cases with distending pain of the breast, add *Radix Salviae Miltiorrhizae* and *Fructus Hordei Germinatus* (30 g) to disperse the stagnated liver – qi and promote blood circulation; for cases with alternating epidsodes of chills and fever, omit *Ligustici Chuanxiong* and add *Radix Scutellariae* and *Herba Artemisiae Annuae* to clear away the gallbladder heat.

3. Also applicable to cases of pleurisy, cholecystitis, mastitis, hyperplasia of mammary gland, etc., which are attributive to stagnation of liver – qi and vital qi.

Decoction of Gentianae for Purging Liver – Fire
(Longdan xie gan tang)

Ingredients

Herba Gentianae	6 g
Radix Bupleuri	6 g
Radix Glycyrrhizae	6 g
Rhizoma Alismatis	10 g
Semen Plantaginis	10 g
Caulis Akebiae	10 g
Radix Rehmanniae	10 g
Fructus Gardeniae	10 g
Radix Scutellariae	10 g
Radix Angelicae Sinensis	3 g

Decoct the above ingredients in a right amount of water for oral administration.

Efficacy

Purging the sthenia fire of liver and gallbladder, clearing away the dampness

— heat evil from triple jiao; mainly for cases with flaming up of sthenia fire in the liver and gallbladder, manifested by headache, hypochondriac pain, bitter taste in the mouth, congestion of the conjunctiva and deafness, and for cases with downward attack of dampness — heat from the liver and gallbladder, manifested by stranguria with turbid urine, pruritus vulvae and leukorrhagia.

Indications

1. For cases of jaundice attributive to dampness — heat attacking the liver and gallbladder, omit *Glycyrrhizae* and *Rehmanniae* and add *Herba Artemisiae Scopariae* and *Radix et Rhizoma Rhei* to eliminate the heat evil through urination and defecation.

2. For cases of leukorrhagia, with yellow or red and white, thick, foul discharge, red tongue with yellowish and greasy fur, smooth and rapid pulse, which are attributive to downward attack of dampness — heat from the liver meridian, omit *Glycyrrhizae* and use *Cortex Phellodendri* instead of *Scutellariae*.

3. Also applicable to cases of acute conjunctivitis, acute otitis media, furuncle of the vestibulum nasi and external auditory canal, hypertension which are attributive to flaming up of sthenia fire in the liver and gallbladder; to cases of icteric hepatitis, cholecystitis, herpes zoster which are attributive to retention of dampness — heat evil in the liver and gallbladder; to cases of urinary infection, pelvic inflammation, prostatitis, which are attributive to downward attack of dampness — heat evil from the liver and gallbladder.

Pulse — Activating Powder
(Sheng mai san)

Ingredients

Radix Ginseng	10 g
Radix Ophiopogonis	15 g
Fructus Schisandrae	6 g

Decoct the above ingredients in a right amount of water for oral administration.

Efficacy

Supplementing qi, promoting the production of body fluid, astringing yin-fluid and arresting sweat.

Indications

Syndrome of impairment of both qi and yin manifested by general debility, shortness of breath, disinclination to talk, thirst with profuse sweat, dry tongue and throat, deficient and weak pulse, or impairment of the lung due to chronic cough, dry cough with shortness of breath, spontaneous perspiration or palpitation, and faint pulse with tendency to exhaustion.

The recipe can be modified to deal with dehydrant shock caused by heat stroke, bleeding, severe vomiting or diarrhea, dramatic injury, scald; or syndrome of impairment of both qi and yin as seen in cases at recovery stage of febrile diseases or at postoperation, or in cases with chronic disorders; or syndrome of deficiency of both qi and yin as seen in such cases as tuberculosis, chronic bronchitis, bronchiectasis, etc..

Cautions

Since it has an astringing effect, it is neither fit for patients whose exopathogen has not been dispelled, nor for those with hyperactivity of heat due to summer-heat diseases, but without impairment of qi and body fluid.

Decoction for Rashes Subsidence
(Hua ban tang)

Ingredients

Gypsum Fibrosum   30 g

Rhizoma Anemarrhenae	12 g
Radix Scrophulariae	10 g
Radix Glycyrrhizae	6 g
Cornu Rhinocerotis	6 g
Semen Oryzae Sativae	20 g

Decoct the above ingredients in a right amount of water for oral administration.

Efficacy

Clearing away heat evil and toxic material, cooling blood and letting tghe rashes subsided; mainly for cases attributive to involvement of qifen and xuefen by severe heat and extravasation of blood - heat, which are manifested by high fever, dark - red rashes, dry mouth, restlessness, or even unconsciousness and delinum, red tongue with yellow fur.

Indications

1. This prescription is applied for cases due to involvement of xuefen by severe heat in qifen, or involvement of both xuefen and qifen by severe heat.

2. Applicable to cases attributive to attack of the stomach by liver - fire with damage of the stomach vessels, which are manifested by hematemesis, irritability, red tongue with yellow fur, wiry and rapid pulse.

3. For cases attributive to hyperactivity of stomach - fire with involvement of blood, which are manifested by tooth bleeding, gingivitis, headache, foul breath, red tongue with yellow fur, bounding and rapid pulse, add *Radix Cyathulae* to let the fire running downward.

4. Also applicable to cses of typnus, erysipelas, epidemic meningitis, septicemia, etc. with fever and skin rashes attributive to involvement of qifen and xuefen by severe heat, or cases of esophageal varicosis with hematemesis attributive to attack of the stomach by liver - fire, or cases of periodontal diseases, necrotizing ulcerative gingivitis with tooth bleeding attributive to hyperactivity of stomach - fire.

Decoction of Restoration
(Fuyuan huoxue tang)

Ingredients

Radix Bupleuri	10 g
Radix Trichosanthis	10 g
Radix Angelicae Sinensis	10 g
Squama Manitis Praeparata	10 g
Radix et Rhizoma Rhei	10 g
Semen Persicae	10 g
Flos Carthami	6 g
Radix Glycyrrhizae	3 g
wine	q.s.

Decoct the above ingredients in a right amount of water for oral administration.

Efficacy

Activating blood circulation, removing blood stasis, dispersing the depressed liver – qi and dredging the passage of meridians; mainly for cases of swelling and pain over the chest and hypochondrium due to trauma.

Indications

1. This is a commonly – used prescription for traumata of chest and hypochondrium with swelling, pain and ecchymoses. For injury of the upper limbs, add *Ramulus Cinnamomi*; for that of the lower limbs, add *Radix Achyranthis Bidentatae*.

2. Also applicable to cases with chest intercostal neuralgia and costal chondritis which are attributive to retention of blood stasis.

Decoction for Severe Phlegm – Heat Syndrome in the Chest
(Da xian xiong tang)

Ingredients

Radix et Rhizoma Rhei	12 g
Natrii Sulfas	10 g
Radix Euphorbiae Kansui (powder, not for decocting)	1.5 g

Decoct the above ingredients in a right amount of water for oral administration.

Efficacy

Purging, eliminating water retention, relieving the accumulation of heat evil; mainly for syndrome attributive to evil accumulating in the thorax, manifested by severe pain and tenderness over the upper abdomen, fever, constipation, sunken and tense pulse, etc..

Indications

1. This prescription is applied for a critical case and should be used as early as possible. Diarrhea usually occurs half an hour after the decoction is taken. One dose may be repeated if diarrhea does not occur after one hour. Overdosage should be prohibited, otherwise the healthy qi may be impaired.

2. Also applicable to cases of acute pancreatitis edematous type, and acute cholecystitis, which are attributive to simultaneous attack of water and heat evil.

Decoction for Soothing the Intestine
(Chang ning tang)

Ingredients

Radix Angelicae Sinensis	15 g

Radix Rehmanniae Praeparata	15 g
Radix Codonopsis Pilosulae	10 g
Radix Ophiopogonis	10 g
Colla Corii Asini	10 g
Rhizoma Dioscoreae	10 g
Radix Dipsaci	10 g
Radix Glycyrrhizae	3 g
Cortex Cinnamomi	1 g

Decoct the above ingredients in a right amount of water for oral administration.

Efficacy

Nourishing blood and benefiting vital qi; mainly for cases of postpartum anemia with dull aching over the lower abdomen which can be relieved by pressing, discharge of scanty thin lochia, dizziness, tinnitus, palpitation, amnesia, pale complexion, constipation, pale tongue, small and weak pulse.

Indications

1. Applicable to cases of metrorrhagia with profuse thin and pale discharge, spiritlessness, dizziness, tinnitus, lumbago, weakness of knees, darkish complexion, pale tongue, sunken and small, weak pulse, which are attributive to impairment of liver and kidney and deficiency of blood and vital qi.

2. Also indicated for cases of ecthyma accompanied with pale tongue, small and rapid pulse, which are attributive to deficiency of blood and vital qi.

3. Also applicable to cases of chronic pelvic inflammation, hypofunction of anterior pituitary, chronic hypoadrenocorticism, dysfunctional uterine bleeding, phlebeurysma of lower limbs, chronic osteomyelitis, which are attributive to deficiency of blood and vital qi.

Decoction of Angelicae Sinensis for Analgesic
(Danggui niantong tang)

Ingredients

Rhizoma seu Radix Notopterygii	10 g
Herba Artemisiae Scopariae	10 g
Radix Ledebouriellae	10 g
Polyporus Umbellatus	10 g
Radix Puerariae	10 g
Rhizoma Atractylodis	10 g
Radix Angelicae Sinensis	12 g
Rhizoma Atractylodis Macrocephalae	12 g
Radix Scutellariae	8 g
Rhizoma Anemarrhenae	8 g
Rhizoma Alismatis	6 g
Rhizoma Cimicifugae	6 g
Radix Codonopsis Pilosulae	6 g
Radix Sophorae Flavescentis	6 g
Radix Glycyrrhizae Praeparata	3 g

Decoct the above ingredients in a right amount of water for oral administration.

Efficacy

Drying dampness, clearing away heat, activating blood circulation and expelling wind, mainly for cases attributive to attack of dampness and heat, which manifest swelling and pain of the joints, fever, aversion to wind, feeling of oppression over the chest, yellow and greasy fur on the tongue, soft and floating, slow or smooth and rapid pulse.

Indications

1. For cases of wet beriberi with oliguira, yellow and greasy fur on the

tongue, soft and floating, slow pulse, which are attributive to retention of dampness – heat in the meridians and stagnation of vital energy and blood, increase the dosage of *Atractylodis* and decrease the dose of *Scutellariae* and *Anemarrhenae*.

2. Also indicated for cases attributive to retention of dampness and toxic material in the muscles and skin, when manifest pyogenic infection of skin, accompanied with fever, thirst, yellow and greasy fur on tongue, soft and floating, slow pulse.

3. Also applicable to cases of rheumatic arthritis, periomarthritis, multiple neuritis, etc. which are attributive to retention of dampness – heat in the meridians; and to cases of impetigo, folliculitis, paronychia, etc. attributive to retention of dampness and toxic material in the muscles and skin.

Decoction of Angelicae Sinensis for Warming Cold Limbs
(Danggui sini tang)

Ingredients

Radix Angelicae Sinensis	10 g
Ramulus Cinnamomi	10 g
Radix Paeoniae Alba	12 g
Herba Asari	6 g
Radix Glycyrrhizae Praeparata	6 g
Caulis Akebiae	6 g
Fructus Ziziphi Jujubae	6 pcs

Decoct the above ingredients in a right amount of water for oral administration.

Efficacy

Warming the channel, expelling cold evil, nourishing blood and dredging the passage of channels; mainly for cases due to deficiency of blood, attack of cold evil and impediment of blood circulation, which are manifested by cold limbs, indistinct pulse, pale tongue with whitish fur.

Indications

1. For cases of dysmenorrhea attributive to deficiency of blood and presence of cold evil, omit *Akebiae* and add *Radix Rehmanniae Praeparata* to nourish the blood and regulate menstruation.

2. For cases with cold colic testalgia referring to the lower abdomen, sunken and wiry pulse, add *Fructus Foeniculi* to warm the liver and regulate vital energy.

4. Also aplicable to cases with cold limbs or abdominal pain occurring in thromboangiitis, *Raynaud*'s disease, acrocyanosis, chilblain, indirect inguinal hernia, dysmenorrhea, etc., which are attributive to blood deficiency and affection of cold evil.

Decoction of Indigo Naturalis for Rashes Subsidence
(Xiaoban qingdan san)

Ingredients

Indigo Naturalis	5 g
Rhizoma coptidis	12 g
Radix Scrophulariae	12 g
Cornu Rhinocerotis	9 g
Rhizoma Anemarrhenae	9 g
Fructus Gardeniae	9 g
Gypsum Fibrosum	30 g
Radix Codonopsis Pilosulae	6 g
Radix Bupleuri	6 g
Radix Glycyrrhizae	3 g
Rhizoma Zingiberis Recens	3 pcs
Fructus Ziziphi Jujubae	2 pcs
vinegar	a spoonful

Decoct the above ingredients in a right amount of water for oral administration.

Efficacy

Purging fire evil, eliminating toxic material, cooling blood and dispersing rashes; mainly for eruptive diseases of yang type attributive to hyperactivity of heat evil at both qifen and yingfen, and extravasation of blood, which are manifested by red rashes over the skin, high fever, irritability, thirst, red tongue with yellow and dry fur, bounding and smooth rapid pulse.

Indications

1. Applicable to cases of hematemesis with bright red or dark purplish bloody discharge, constipation or blackish stools, red tongue with yellow and dry fur, smooth and rapid pulse, which are attributive to damage of the stomach collateral by heat, and adverse rising of vital qi and fire.

2. For cases of burn manifested by local erythema, pain and heat, accompanied with high fever, irritability, thirst, constipation, red tongue with yellow and dry fur, bounding and rapid pulse, which are attributive to inward attack of potent fire evil and hyperactivity of heat at both qifen and yingfen, *Radix Ginseng* or *Radix panacis Quinquefolii* is used instead of *Codonopsis Pilosulae*.

3. Also applicable to cases of scarlet fever, dengue fever, typhus fever, erysipelas, exudative erythema multiforme, etc. with red eruptions and high fever, which are attributive to hyperactivity of heat at both qifen and yingfen, and extravasation of blood; also to cases of rupture of which are attributive to damage of stomach collateral by heat and adverse rising of vital qi and fire.

Chapter Twenty-one

Decoction of Sargassum for Goiter
(Haizao yuhu tang)

Ingredients

Sargassum	9 g
Thallus Laminariae seu Eckloniae	9 g
Thallus Laminariae Japonicae	9 g
Rhizoma Pinelliae	9 g
Fructus Forsythiae	9 g
Bulbus Fritillariae Thunbergii	9 g
Radix Angelicae Sinensis	9 g
Radix Angelicae Pubescentis	6 g
Pericarpium Citri Reticulatae	6 g
Rhizoma Ligustici Chuanxiong	6 g
Exocarpium Citri Grandis	6 g
Radix Glycyrrhizae	3 g

Decoct the above ingredients in a right amount of water for oral administration.

Efficacy

Dispersing phlegm, softening masses, regulating qi and dispelling stagnation; mainly for goiter attributive to stagnation of phlegm and qi, which is round, soft, smooth and slowly growing, with wiry pulse.

Indications

1. For scrofula attributive to stagnation of phlegm and vital qi, which are hard and movable, accompanied with wiry and smooth pulse, omit *Angelicae Pubescentis* from the prescription.

2. Indicated for hard, movable and slow-growing masses of the breast, accompanied with wiry pulse, which are attributive to the stagnation of phlegm and vital qi.

3. Also applicable to adenoma of thyroid, nodular goiter, thyroiditis, cervical lymphadenitis, fibrodenoma and cystic hyperplasia of the breast.

Pill for Eliminating Phlegm Evil
(Gun Tan Wan)

INGREDIENTS

Radix et Rhizoma Rhei	240 g
Radix Scutellariae	240 g
Lignum Aquilariae Resinatum	15 g
Lapis Chloriti	30 g

EFFICACY

Purging fire and eliminating phlegm; mainly for cases of chronic phlegm – syndrome of sthenic heat type, manifested by mania with frigthening, or dyspneic cough with thick sputum, or feeling of oppression over the chest and epigastrium, or dizziness with profuse expectoration, constipationm, yellow and thick, greasy fur on the tongue, smooth and rapid, strong pulse.

INDICATIONS

1. This formula cannot be taken as decoction.
2. Applicable to cases of nasosinusitis manifested by stuffy nose, headache, turbid, foul, thick and yellow nasal discharge, yellow and greasy fur on the tongue, wiry and rapid pulse, which are attributive to the attack of phlegm – heat from the spleen and stomach to the nasal orifice.
3. Applicable to cases of chronic suppurative otitis media accompanied with deafness, tinnitus, yellow and greasy fur on the tongue, wiry and rapid pulse, which are attributive to the attack of dampness – heat of lvier and gallbladder to the orifice.
4. Applicable to cases of schizophrenia, manic – depressive psychosis,

chronic bronchitis, emphysema, etc., which are attributive to chronic phlegm-syndrome of sthenic heat type.

图书在版编目(CIP)数据

中医治疗男性病:英文./侯景伦主编.
- 北京:学苑出版社,1997.
ISBN7-5077-1339-3

Ⅰ.中… Ⅱ.①侯… Ⅲ.①男性生殖器疾病-中医治疗法-英文 Ⅳ.R277.57

中国版本图书馆CIP数据核字(97)第09796号

中医治疗男性病

主编 侯景伦

编委 赵 昕 李国华

学苑出版社出版
(中国北京万寿路西街11号)
邮政编码 100036
北京大兴沙窝店印刷厂印刷
中国国际图书贸易总公司发行
(中国北京车公庄西路35号)
北京邮政信箱第399号 邮政编码100044
英文版 16开本
1997年5月第1版第1次印刷
ISBN7-5077-1339-3

08900
14-E-3130P